P9-DMD-977

THE ELEPHANT MAN

THE
ELEPHANT
MAN

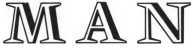

Frederick Drimmer

illustrated with photographs

G. P. Putnam's Sons
New York

Photographs on pages 2, 5, 6, 7, 8, 9, 10, 11 and 12 of
the photographic section were kindly supplied by
the London Hospital Medical College Museum.

Library of Congress Cataloging in Publication Data
Drimmer, Frederick
The elephant man.
Bibliography: p.
Summary: Traces the history of Joseph Merrick, called
the Elephant Man because of a deformity, from his birth in
central England to his death in a London hospital in 1890.
1. Merrick, Joseph Carey, 1862 or 3–1890.
2. Neurofibromatosis—Patients—England—Biography.
3. Abnormalities, Human—Patients—England—Biography.
[1. Merrick, Joseph Carey, 1862 or 3–1890. 2. Neuro-
fibromatosis. 3. Physically handicapped] I. Title.
RC280.N4D75   1985   362.1'9699283'00924 [B] [92] 84-26583

ISBN 0-399-21262-0
Third Impression

for Andrew and Amelia

Acknowledgments

It is a delight, not a duty, to make acknowledgment of the help and encouragement generously afforded me when I was planning and carrying out this project.

To Refna Wilkin, my editor, I owe a singular debt of gratitude for her interest, enthusiastic support, and perceptive suggestions along the way.

Of considerable value were the advice and information provided by Percy G. Nunn, assistant curator of the London Hospital Medical College Museum, where the skeleton and memorabilia of Joseph Carey Merrick are preserved. Mr. Nunn, an authority on the Elephant Man, patiently took time out from his busy day to explain the physical peculiarities of Merrick's condition and supplied answers to my questions with insight and unfailing courtesy. He also made photographs available.

Of great assistance was the staff of the National Neurofibromatosis Foundation in New York City. They provided me with highly useful, authoritative information about the nature of NF, the response of patients to the disorder, and how it is treated. Felice Yahr, the executive director, was kind enough to review my Afterword and provide helpful suggestions.

In my search for information I have repeatedly had occasion to make use of the resources of a number of fine libraries—in particular the libraries of the Royal College of Surgeons and the British Library in London; the Academy of Medicine and the Research Libraries of New York City; and, in Connecticut, the Wiggans Library of Norwalk Hospital (Jean Botts, librarian) as well as the public libraries of Norwalk, Westport, and Wilton, and the library of Yale University Medical College in New Haven.

For providing firsthand information about animal behavior I am indebted to John Iaderosa, zoologist, of the New York Zoological Society.

Gaby Monet of Concepts Unlimited, Inc., New York, made available illustrations relating to the Elephant Man from the television motion picture *Some Call Them Freaks* (Home Box Office), which she produced and directed.

I am under an obligation to Evelyn Drimmer, my wife, for her patient review of the manuscript and her many invaluable suggestions, and to my children, John and Jean, for their encouragement.

I should not fail to acknowledge my deep debt to the late Sir Frederick Treves, who first brought Joseph Merrick to the attention of medical science and immortalized him in the sensitive account in his *The Elephant Man and Other Reminiscences*. This account I included in my book *Very Special People*.

Indispensable knowledge and clues were provided by the British authors Dr. Michael Howell and Peter Ford. Their book *The True History of the Elephant Man* is a classic work of research as well as the standard authority on the subject. Ashley Montagu, in *The Elephant Man: A Study in Human Dignity*, also gave me significant insights.

Contents

As a specimen of humanity,
Merrick was ignoble and repulsive;
but the spirit of Merrick,
if it could be seen
in the form of the living,
would assume the figure
of an upstanding and heroic man,
smooth browed and clean of limb,
and with eyes that flashed
undaunted courage.

—SIR FREDERICK TREVES

THE ELEPHANT MAN

ONE

Man Into Animal

How could the young surgeon possibly guess, that gray November morning, that the most remarkable adventure of his life was about to begin?

For Frederick Treves the day started out almost like any other. Up at five, he worked in his chilly study, keeping close to the blazing fireplace to stay warm. Almost before he knew it, the grandfather clock in the corner struck eight. Time to go to the hospital, he thought. Kissing his pretty wife and two little daughters goodbye, he hurried out and hailed a hansom cab.

The day was raw and blustery. The wind with frosty fingers snatched at men's hats and rattled signs hanging over shop windows. White clouds of mist exploded from the nostrils of the horse pulling Treves's cab as the driver cracked his whip. Dark clouds, threatening rain, raced across the sky.

Bouncing over the cobblestones, the cab swung through a wide gateway and pulled up in front of the London Hospital. The enormous red brick building, with its hundreds of beds, was the biggest hospital of its kind in the British Empire. It was also the busiest, and patients would already be lined up waiting for Treves.

13

The tall, broad-shouldered surgeon sprinted up the steps, waved to the nurses in their starchy aprons in the lobby, and walked rapidly into the dressing room.

"Good morning, Mr. Treves! Good morning, Mr. Treves!" a dozen voices sang out—the voices of his students and two nurses. Eager hands took his overcoat, his jacket, and his top hat and helped him into his long white surgical coat.

Treves scrubbed his hands briskly with soap and water. "All right, Nurse, bring on the first patient."

The dressing room was the place where the emergency cases were brought. Into this room, each day, came or were carried people young and old who had been maimed and mangled in every imaginable kind of accident—and some you might find hard to imagine.

The London Hospital was in the East End, one of the ugliest, most crowded sections of the great city. The air was foul with the smoke of countless chimneys. Walk down the streets and you could hear the pounding and clattering of sewing machines as women slaved from dawn until late into the night to earn a bare living. You could hear the chatter of foreign tongues—Russian, French, German, Spanish, Indian, Chinese, African, and many others. The East End was home to poor immigrants from every land. They lived packed close together in rat-plagued, dingy tenements—whole families in a single room—and worked long, hard hours at home or in warehouses and sweatshops and on the docks in the area.

More people seemed to get hurt in the East End than almost anywhere else in the vast city. How lucky it was for the victims that the London Hospital happened to be so close by!

London in 1884—the year Frederick Treves's great adventure began—had few ambulances to whisk accident victims quickly and safely to the hospital. If a cart or a cab wasn't handy, it was up to good-hearted people to get them there. When someone was injured in a factory or in the streets, fellow workers or kindly passersby would take down a shutter from a window and use it as a stretcher. Or they might carry the victim by hand, as carefully as they were able, like a package that was coming apart. Two workmen would hold the victim's legs, others each arm, and another, walking backward, would hold the person's head. In this way they would bear the victim through the swarming, noisy streets until they came to the Whitechapel Road, where the London Hospital stood (and still stands today). In the bustling lobby a nurse would take one look and wave the bearers and the injured person to the dressing rooms, one for the women and another for the men.

It was a lucky patient who opened his eyes to see the handsome face of young Surgeon Treves looking thoughtfully down at him. Treves always seemed to know at once just what needed to be done, and he did it swiftly and deftly, with hands that were strong and steady.

Frederick Treves was no ordinary surgeon. Only thirty-one, he had been working as a surgeon for nine years, and had already written an important textbook on surgical anatomy. He knew more about the human body and how to set it right when it was injured or diseased than many medical men twice his age. He had performed hundreds and hundreds of operations, and he was always looking for ways to make them better, safer, and more comfortable for the patient. The London Hospital had its own medical college, where Treves lectured on anatomy to classes that were always jammed.

One after another, patients took their place on the big black couch in Treves's dressing room. Some were unconscious, others groaning in pain or delirious. A man who had been run over by a wagon had the red ends of his broken legbones sticking out of his torn trousers. A boy (children worked in factories in those days) had had his arm smashed by a machine, and black grease dripped from him with his blood. The throat of a man had been cut and he was gasping for breath. There were other cases just as serious. For the rest of their lives, they would remember the surgeon's cool, gentle fingers, his warm, friendly smile, and his reassuring words as he cleansed and stitched up their wounds or set their broken bones. To Frederick Treves, dedicated surgeon and healer, the life and feelings of the poorest of his patients were as precious as those of the richest and most powerful in the land.

As Treves worked, his students formed a tight circle around him and the patient. They studied every move the surgeon made and they listened intently. Treves was explaining just what he was doing and why he was doing it, and they didn't want to miss one word, one action. When he asked any of them to assist him, they stepped forward at once, eager and pleased. Many had enrolled in the London Hospital's medical college just because they knew Frederick Treves was on the staff and he would be their teacher.

The long black hands of the clock were reaching toward noon.

"That's all for this morning, gentlemen," said Treves, and he stooped over the basin to scrub his hands. The long white coat that had looked so fresh and clean when he had put it on was wrinkled and stained now and it was stiff with dry blood. One of the students quickly helped him out of it, while another stood ready with the surgeon's jacket and another with his overcoat and top hat.

Waving a lively goodbye, Treves stepped briskly out into the street. Usually he took a cab home at this time for a quick lunch with his wife. He had many private patients, and they would soon be crowding not only his waiting room but almost every other room of the house on Wimpole Street. Today, however, he was skipping lunch. He had somewhere special to go.

Only the day before, his assistant, Dr. Reginald Tuckett, had told him about an unusual show he had seen on the Whitechapel Road.

"It's a freak, Freddie, but what a freak! They call him the Elephant Man. This chap is so bizarre I can't begin to tell you what he looks like. I know you're keen about that kind of thing. Why don't you go and see him for yourself before the show moves on?"

His assistant knew him well; Treves did have a boundless curiosity about anything offbeat or unusual in his field. A rare, unexplained disease, a strange and difficult medical case meant more than meat and drink to him. Tuckett had given him the address of the shop where the freak could be seen, and that was where he was heading at this moment.

The black clouds had disappeared and the sun was shining brightly. Pausing on the curb, Treves waited for a van to pass and then he plunged into the heavy traffic like a swimmer into a swift-moving stream. On the other side, peddlers and their carts jammed the sidewalk. He moved quickly past them to the row of shops that lined the street.

It didn't take Treves long to find the number he was looking for, 123 Whitechapel Road. It was almost directly opposite the hospital entrance, and he knew he had found it even before he saw the number.

Covering all of the shopfront except the door was a large canvas sheet with a picture on it. The colors were harsh and bright and it was crudely painted, but the surgeon would remember it to his dying day.

It was a picture right out of a nightmare.

Against a background of tall, green-leaved palm trees, Treves saw one of the most frightful figures he had ever seen. It was a man, but a man only in part, for he was in the process of turning into something else—into an animal. The figure was naked except for a cloth about the middle. Most of the body seemed normal enough as far down as the knees. Below the knees, however, the legs were unnaturally broad and heavy, and they were colored gray, like an elephant's. One of the arms was not an arm at all but the gray leg of an elephant.

It was the head that Treves found most troubling. It too was gray, and enormous and domed, like the head of an elephant. Out of the mouth grew two small, stubby yellow tusks. The nose was larger and much longer than a man's and it twisted upward and back—like the trunk of an elephant trumpeting in anger.

Only the eyes seemed fully human. They gazed out of the elephant-head with what, Treves thought, was a look of unspeakable horror.

TWO

Freak Show

SEE THE ELEPHANT MAN!" the sign over the shopfront shouted in bright red letters. "ONLY TWOPENCE."

Treves went to the door and grasped the knob firmly. He turned it but the door didn't open. He pushed it and pulled it. Still the door refused to budge. He peered through the glass but it was so dirty he could see nothing; or perhaps that was because it was so dim and dark inside.

He rapped sharply on the glass and waited. No one came to open up.

"Want to go in, guv'nor? Want to see the Elephant Man?" piped a high, eager little voice beside him.

Treves looked down into the face of a small boy in a torn sweater who was blowing on cold white fingers. "Yes, my lad, I do. Where is the manager?"

The boy raised an imaginary glass to his lips and pretended to take a sip. He winked. "Down the road a bit at the pub, takin' a drop. Want me to fetch 'im for you, guv'nor?"

Treves took out a copper. It disappeared as if by magic into the

18

boy's pocket. Turning, he shot down the street and vanished into the nearest pub. A minute or two later he came shooting back.

Out of the pub stepped a slender little man wearing a flashy checked coat and a curly-brimmed bowler hat. He saw Treves standing in front of the shop and waved a silvery cane as if to tell him to wait. Then he hurried forward.

"Good day, sir." The little man raised his bowler hat and bowed. Treves noticed he was wearing white gloves—and on the fingers of the gloves he had heavy rings with big flashy stones. "Want to see the Elephant Man, do we? Great sight he is, too." He unbuttoned his coat and reached into his vest pocket for a key. Rows of chains were strung across his vest, and silver coins jingled on them.

The little man found the key and looked up at the tall surgeon. "Seeing as this is to be a private showing there'll have to be an—ahem!—extra charge."

"I understand. Will this be enough?" A new shilling piece sparkled between Treves's fingers.

"Just right, guv'nor, just right." The key grated in the rusty lock. "Step this way, sir."

Treves walked before him into the shop. Inside it felt almost as cold as on the street. It was quite dark because of the big sign that covered the window in front. The place was dank and dusty. A curious, unpleasant odor that Treves couldn't identify filled the air.

But where was the Elephant Man?

Toward the rear Treves saw a red curtain suspended by rings from a cord strung across the shop. The flashy little man took up a position at one end of the curtain. He bared his yellow teeth in a smile and jingled the silver coins on his vest chains.

"Behind this curtain, guv'nor, is the one and only Elephant Man—the Eighth Wonder of the World." He stabbed at the air with his silvery cane as if he were cutting his words into it. "Half an elephant and half a man, that's what he is. You've never seen his like before and you never will again.

"You know that when a woman is pregnant and something frightens her it can leave a lasting mark on her baby. If a mouse runs out in front of her and she claps her hand to her cheek in terror, her poor babe could be born with a birthmark on its cheek in the shape of a mouse. If she's scared by a monkey she could have a babe all covered with hair. Or it might be very tiny, even a midget. *

"The mother of this strange creature was frightened by an elephant. Almost trampled her, it did. After her baby was born she saw, to her horror, that the poor little tyke was no normal infant. He was part elephant and part human. The unhappy woman almost died of the shock."

The showman cut into the air again with his cane. "The Elephant Man has been brought to London at considerable expense so you can see this great mistake of Mother Nature. Is he a man? Is he a beast? Now, sir, you will be able to decide for yourself." He took hold of one end of the red curtain. "Behold, the extraordinary ELEPHANT MAN!" And with a triumphant swing of his arm he pulled the curtain aside.

In the darkness at the rear of the shop the first thing Treves noticed was a faint blue light. It came from a gas jet heating a large brick on a tripod. Directly behind it, on a low stool, crouched an odd figure wrapped almost completely in a brown blanket. The figure didn't stir when the curtain was drawn, but sat hunched over the flame, as close to it as possible.

Huddled in the gloom, lit only by the tiny glow of the flame, the creature seemed to Treves the loneliest, most solitary being he had ever seen. It could have been, he thought, a captive chained in a cavern . . . or perhaps a wizard watching for something magical to spring out of the ghostly flame. Yet just outside the window of the shop the sun was shining cheerfully and the busy world of the

---

*This belief was widely held at the time by both medical men and the general public. Naturally, when a baby was born with any unusual mark or deformity it was easy to think back and find something that had happened to the pregnant woman that could explain the peculiarity. Nowadays we know birth abnormalities are genetic or due to medication, disease, or other physical causes.

Whitechapel Road was going about its business. Treves could hear the footsteps of people passing by, the whistling of a delivery boy, the familiar clatter of horses' hooves in the road.

"Stand up!" the showman called gruffly, like an animal trainer giving a command to a beast in a cage.

Slowly the thing raised itself from the stool. The blanket that covered its head and back slipped to the dusty floor and the creature stood trembling in the cold.

The Elephant Man was naked to the waist. A pair of shabby, overlarge trousers covered his bottom half, trousers that had once belonged to some gentleman's dress suit. His feet were bare.

To Frederick Treves, the surgeon, hideously deformed or mangled faces and bodies were no novelty. He saw them every day on the operating table and in the wards of the London Hospital. Never in his entire life, however, had he seen anyone who looked as terrible as the creature that now stood before him.

From the large size of the figure in the painting on the front of the shop, Treves had expected the Elephant Man would be a giant. Instead, he was slight and quite short, just a little more than five feet tall. Because his back was bent and bowed he looked even shorter.

Nothing about the Elephant Man was more shocking than his head. It was enormous, and deformed with lumps of bone and growths of spongy skin. On the forehead a great mass of bone stood out like a loaf, almost hiding his right eye. Scraggly locks of brown hair covered the top of his head, except where outgrowths of flesh took their place.

The Elephant Man's mouth was a twisted, slobbering gash. From the upper jaw a mass of bone stuck out like a pink tusk, turning the lip inside out. Perhaps it was because of this pink stump that he was called the Elephant Man. His nose, however, was nothing like an elephant's trunk. A shapeless chunk of flesh, you knew it was a nose only because it was set below his eyes and above his mouth. The face showed as much expression as the gnarled trunk of an old tree.

His thumbs in his vest pockets, the little showman jingled the silver coins once more. "About face!" he commanded.

21

The Elephant Man nodded and swung slowly around, limping as he moved. From the rear he presented almost as gruesome a sight as he did in front. Huge masses of thick, spongy skin hung from his back like bags. They looked like cauliflower covered with brownish or purplish rot. Another bag of spongy brown flesh the size of a teacup hung from the back of his head. Another, hanging from the chest in front, looked like the dewlap of a lizard.

On the painting outside the shop the creature's right arm had appeared big and heavy, and gray as an elephant's hide. The real arm was nothing like that but it was horrible enough. Shapeless and much larger than an ordinary arm, it too was covered with loose brown skin. The hand was big and clumsy; the thumb was like a radish, the fingers like thick roots. The palm and the back were exactly the same, so it looked more like a paddle than a hand. How much could the Elephant Man possibly do with an arm and a hand like that?

The left arm was completely different. Its shape was perfect and it was covered by fine skin. Treves bent over to see it better. It was so beautiful he decided it should have belonged to a woman rather than a man.

The Elephant Man's feet, however, were as bad as anything Treves had ever seen. They were so misshapen and swollen, no ordinary shoes could possibly fit on them.

"Walk!" thundered the showman, as if he was giving an order to some great half-wild beast of the jungle.

The little man bent over toward his stool, where a cane rested. He picked it up with his good hand, which seemed to be shaking with the cold. Then, leaning heavily upon the cane, he dragged himself forward. After a few steps he turned around and hobbled back. His movements were painful and clumsy and he swayed from side to side. Treves's diagnostic eye could see he had once had a bad disease of the hip.

"Say a few words for the gentleman."

The Elephant Man turned awkwardly about to face Treves and the showman. High-pitched flutelike sounds came from his twisted mouth. So distorted were his words by the mass of bone growing from his jaw that Treves could understand little of what the pitiful creature said. He thought he recognized the words "Thank you."

Poor chap! the surgeon thought. He has more than one man's share of the ills of this world.

Ever since Treves had entered the shop he had been aware of a peculiar, sickening smell in the air. When he stood close to the Elephant Man he found it was much more powerful. It came, he decided, from the ugly bags of skin hanging from the body. The smell was so unpleasant that the surgeon had to hold his handkerchief to his nose.

The Elephant Man straightened up now, holding himself as erect as his twisted body would allow. He bowed stiffly at the waist. The show was over.

Hobbling back to his stool, he laid down his cane, pulled his blanket over his head and shoulders, and sat down. He drew as close to the little flame and the hot brick as he could. Now he looked exactly as he did when Treves had first set eyes on him—isolated, withdrawn, the picture of loneliness.

The surgeon placed his hand on the showman's shoulder. "I have a special interest in this fellow. I'm a surgeon. Frederick Treves, lecturer in anatomy at the London Hospital Medical College across the road."

"Pleased to make your acquaintance, guv'nor. My name's Tom Norman. I exhibit freaks. Midgets, giants, bearded ladies—the whole bloomin' lot. But never have I had a freak like the Elephant Man."

"What can you tell me about him? What's his name? Where does he come from?"

"Name is Joseph Merrick. He's from Leicester."

"I'd like to examine your Elephant Man more closely—in my study at the college. Do you think I could borrow him for an hour or two—at ten tomorrow morning?"

Norman's eyes narrowed. "Can't rightly say. There may be some blokes comin' in here as will want to see him."

"I understand." Treves held out five shillings. "Will this cover your loss?"

"It could, Mr. Treves, it could." The money disappeared into a pocket of the flashy suit. "There's just one problem."

The problem, Norman explained, was that the Elephant Man didn't dare to show himself in the streets of London. He was such a peculiar sight that he attracted a crowd wherever he appeared. The crowd would draw the police, and they would very likely take him off to the police station.

"The only way the poor bloke can appear in public is to wear a disguise," Norman said. He moved toward a dark corner and returned with several objects. "Never seen anything like these, I'll bet."

In one hand Norman held up a black cap. It was huge, as it would have to be to fit the Elephant Man's big domed head. From the front of the cap hung a sort of curtain of brown flannel.

"Like a mask it is," Norman continued. "It hides his whole bloomin' face." The showman thrust his fingers at the flannel. Treves saw them pass through a slit cut across the cloth. "He can see through this," Norman said, "but no one can see him."

The showman next held up a black cape. "Almost the size of a tent, ain't it? Reaches down to the ground so it hides every bloomin' bit of him. . . . And look at these." In his hand he held a pair of great baglike slippers, which Merrick used to cover his deformed feet.

"But," Norman went on, "even in this outfit the poor bloke can't get very far. Just you imagine the crowd he'll collect if he limps across Whitechapel Road in it. There'll be a bloody riot. No, sir, no, sir. Best thing would be to send him over in a cab."

"You're right, man." Treves laid a coin in Norman's palm.

"Right-o." The showman beamed. "He'll be there at ten. Guaranteed."

"Oh, Merrick will need something to show to the guards at the gate so they'll let him in." Treves turned to the Elephant Man. The monstrous face was gazing up at him. It was completely without expression; Treves couldn't tell whether he had been listening or not. "Here's my card, Merrick. Just show it at the gate."

Not a sound came from the Elephant Man's deformed mouth. He simply looked down at the small slip of cardboard Treves had placed in his good hand.

Does he understand? Treves wondered. Perhaps he's retarded.

"Don't worry, sir," Norman reassured. "He'll be there."

"Very good. See you tomorrow at ten," Treves reminded the Elephant Man, patting him on the shoulder. "Thank you, Norman." He turned to go, with the little showman at his heels.

The Elephant Man watched them disappear through the doorway. The key turned in the lock and he was alone again in the silence and the gloom.

A shiver ran through him and he moved closer to the tiny flame. His great head bent over, he stared at the card cradled in his hand.

A half hour later he was still gazing down at it.

THREE

Medical Mystery

I nsistent knuckles rapped at the heavy oaken door of Treves's study at the London Hospital Medical College.

Ten o'clock. He'd been expecting the interruption. "Come in," he called, looking up from the notes on his desk.

The door creaked open. Outside stood the trim capped and aproned figure of Nurse Ireland.

"A visitor for you, Mr. Treves." Her blue eyes rolled back in her head. It was her way of telling him she found his caller very much out of the ordinary.

He grinned. "Show the gentleman in, Nurse. We don't want to keep him waiting, do we?"

She stepped aside. Outlined in the sunlit corridor stood a short figure dressed in a peaked cap and a long black cloak that swept the floor. Bright eyes flickered nervously behind the opening in the brown flannel mask.

"Good morning, Merrick." Treves waved him in.

The shrouded figure lurched forward awkwardly, leaning on a cane. Nurse Ireland, all curiosity, followed briskly.

"Thank you very much, Nurse," Treves dismissed her.

Unwillingly she backed out, pulling the door slowly shut behind her.

"Come, man, give me your hat and cloak and sit here by the fire."

The shock of seeing the monstrous face again made Treves start. He recovered himself at once. "It's a cold day. What would you say to a cup of tea and a bun?"

From Merrick's swollen mouth came the same flutelike sounds Treves had heard the day before. They sounded more like the twittering of a bird than the speech of a human being. He couldn't make out the words but he knew his offer had been accepted.

Holding the cup with his left hand, the Elephant Man lifted the steaming liquid to his thick lips and swallowed. Treves was struck by the delicacy of the hand and the skillful, almost genteel way it manipulated the cup. Even the ugliest of us has some beauty in him, he thought.

The surgeon dipped his pen in the inkwell. "Merrick, are there any others in your family who have this . . . ah . . . condition?"

The Elephant Man stared back at him, wordless.

Poor fellow, he doesn't understand, thought Treves. He did seem slow yesterday in the shop. In his case that's a blessing. How awful it would be if he had all his wits and realized what he is . . . so terribly deformed that anyone who meets him draws back in fright or loathing.

But the Elephant Man must finally have grasped the surgeon's question. The domed head swung heavily from side to side. It looked so massive Treves marveled that the creature could hold it upright on his frail neck.

"Parents living?"

The Elephant Man blinked. Again the musical sounds, as if a bird was in the room. A few words Treves could make out. But most were blurred by the mass of pink bone disfiguring his mouth.

"I'm afraid I don't quite follow you, Merrick."

Again and again Treves repeated his question. Merrick's mother, he gathered at last, was long dead. The Elephant Man wanted to

talk on about her, but Treves was having too much trouble understanding; he had to cut him short. Merrick's father was still among
the living. Did the surgeon imagine it—or was the little man
reluctant to talk about him?

"How old are you?"

The nightmare of a face gazed back at him in silence.

The fellow didn't even know how old he was! Treves couldn't
believe it. He prodded Merrick. But it soon became clear the little
man actually did not know the year he was born. He supposed he
was twenty-two or twenty-three. Treves thought of his two pretty
little daughters. They wouldn't have any trouble remembering their
age—even the baby, who was only two. But in his daughters' case,
he suddenly realized, birthdays were such happy times. . . .

"How long have you had this condition?"

Since early childhood, Merrick seemed to say. As far back as he
could remember, he'd been burdened with the gigantic head, the
big deformed right arm and leg, the misshapen feet. The fearsome
outgrowths of bone, skin, and ill-smelling flesh—he thought they
had come later.

Bit by bit the Elephant Man's sad history was drawn out of him.
Treves had to question the little man time and again and piece
together the sounds he uttered in order to make sense of them. It
was like listening to someone speaking a foreign language in which
you understood only a handful of words.

With his whole heart and soul the Elephant Man believed his
condition was the result of a tragic accident involving his mother. A
little before he was born she'd been in the street, in a crowd
watching a circus parade of animals and showpeople. The crowd
surged forward. The mother-to-be, standing in front, found herself
pushed into the road, under the feet of an elephant. She wasn't hurt
but she was nearly frightened to death. Some time after her baby
was born he began to show the marks of her terrifying experience.
He developed an arm as big as an elephant's leg. A head domed like
an elephant's. And later this warty, elephant-like skin. And . . .

The Elephant Man babbled on and on, almost incoherently.

Treves made no effort to stop him. To Merrick, he saw, the incident was the beginning of all his misfortunes. Telling the story to a sympathetic listener gave him emotional release—and renewed courage to face his bitter fate.

Finally the little man seemed all talked out. Exhausted, he leaned forward in the chair and held his great head in his hands. His shoulders shook with silent sobs.

"Merrick, would you be good enough to take your clothes off? I need to give you a complete physical."

Merrick began to remove his jacket. The surgeon watched the malformed body twist and turn, slowly working itself out of the oversized garment. Treves reached forward to help. But the Elephant Man raised his good hand and waved him off.

"And do it yourself you shall, my lad," said Treves with a grin.

At length Merrick stood bare to the waist, just as the surgeon had seen him the day before.

"Come, come, take off the rest of your things. I really must examine all of you if I'm to be of any help."

Merrick grimaced. He sat down on a chair and writhed his way out of his remaining garments. At last he stood mother-naked in front of the surgeon. To keep his balance he held on to the back of the chair.

If Treves had been disturbed by what he'd seen by the poor light in the shop, he was even more dismayed by what he saw now. Much of Merrick's body was covered with loose warty skin that could be drawn up in immense folds. Big warty flaps of flesh hung from some parts. One flap reached from the buttocks down to the middle of the thigh. It was so thick and extensive, at first Treves thought it was the buttock itself.

By the bright light of his oil lamp, Treves examined the Elephant Man's legs and feet. They had patches large and small of the same warty skin. Below the knees both of the legs were severely misshapen. The toes were the biggest Treves had ever seen. With his sensitive surgeon's fingers he pressed gently down on the thick, rough tissue of the oversized feet and felt the bones beneath. They were abnormally large too.* Standing, Merrick held his left leg in front of him in a stiff, unnatural way, with the heel raised. It was, Treves had observed the day before, the result of an old hip disease. The left foot was almost clubbed.

Treves picked up his tape measure. The little man was only five feet two inches high. His astonishing head, at its widest point, was a good three feet in circumference—the same measurement as his waist! The cranium was completely unsymmetrical. On top of it a great ridge ran from the front to the back of the skull, where it lost itself in lumps of bone of different sizes. Bony tumors as big as tangerines thrust out from the back and side. But these were small in contrast to the bony mass on his forehead. It was so big it overshadowed the right eye. On the right side of the head a lump thrust out so far it made the ear fold over.

The big right arm was three times the size of the left. The wrist was an incredible twelve inches around. The biggest of the fingers of the giant right hand measured five inches around.

"Open wide," said the surgeon. He peered into the red cavern of the Elephant Man's mouth. The bony overgrowth of the upper jaw twisted the mouth out of shape and pushed the nose out of position. The teeth in the distorted jaw were turned and twisted or they weren't where they should have been. Treves discovered a large scar inside the mouth and asked about it. Haltingly the Elephant Man told him a surgeon had cut away a tumor growing there after it got so big it interfered with his eating.

Although Treves was a young man, he was one of the best surgeons in the biggest general hospital in all Britain. He had seen more of the ills and injuries of the human body than most medical

*If Treves had encountered the Elephant Man some years later he could have determined the state of his patient's bones not by feel but by taking X rays. However, in 1884, the date of this incident, the principle of the X ray was still unknown. That was to be discovered in 1895 by the German scientist Wilhelm Conrad Roentgen (1845–1923).

men. But the like of Merrick's disease he had never seen before or even read about. From a surgical point of view—or from any other—the case appeared untreatable.

If only there were something he could do to help the poor chap!

Treves pointed to a large camera on a tripod at one side of the study. The hospital had a medical photographer. Treves himself often painted watercolors of unusual cases in order to round out his records. But for a complicated case like this one the big black box could do the job faster and better than any artist.

"Merrick, I'll need a few photographs of you for my records—and to show to other surgeons."

Merrick's shoulders twisted in a grotesque shrug. He limped forward until he was standing in front of the camera.

"Wrap this around your middle."

Painstakingly the Elephant Man wrapped the towel about his loins while Treves went out. He returned promptly with the hospital photographer, who stopped abruptly when he saw Merrick. Recovering himself, he walked to the camera.

"Merrick, would you be good enough to stand like this?" Treves took a position halfway between full face and profile—what is called a three-quarter view.

The little man studied the pose. He tried to copy it.

Standing behind the camera, the photographer nodded his approval. Treves went back and looked into the viewing field. The deformed right arm, turned toward the lens, loomed gigantic, hanging down as far as the knee. His left arm looked hardly bigger than a child's. The bulging right side of the cranium, the awful legs, the almost clubbed foot—it all showed perfectly.

With a thoughtful expression on his misfortune of a face, the Elephant Man stood patiently, like a model posing for a painting. In spite of his horrible deformities, Treves found a curious grace in the man and his pose.

"Steady!" called the photographer. He pressed the bulb.

The photographer changed the plate. At Treves's command

31

Merrick turned this way and that, taking other positions so his peculiarities could be photographed from different angles. He was as obedient as a small boy.

"Merrick, would you turn about and drop the towel?"

The white cloth fell to the floor. The whole frightful back was exposed, with its covering of fungus-like flesh spreading down to the middle of the thighs like an evil garment designed by some demon. The photographer squeezed the bulb. Treves was pleased, not only with the completeness of the photographic record but with the subject. Merrick, although severely disabled, was far from the imbecile his handicaps had caused the surgeon to believe him at first.

The photographer carried the exposed plates out of the room. Treves sat down at his desk and began to write. Merrick struggled back into his clothes. Lurching over to the surgeon's desk, he lowered himself into the chair beside it. He cocked his head to one side. Treves heard the birdlike sounds again.

"I suppose you want to know what I make of your condition. Not much, I'm afraid. Your case is completely outside my experience. It's what we call a congenital disorder—something you were born with. But that's not telling you anything you don't know."

Merrick took a deep breath. He nodded sadly.

"I'm going to follow up on your case," continued Treves. "In a few weeks there'll be a meeting of the Pathological Society of London. Medical men who specialize in all different kinds of diseases will be there. I want you to be present too so I can put your case to them as clearly as possible. Someone may come up with a treatment that may be helpful. What do you say?"

Merrick made no reply. I suppose, thought Treves, he's heard the same story so many times before that another vague promise can't get much of a rise out of him. But at least he hasn't said no.

The surgeon leaned over and patted the little man on the shoulder. "Where there's life there's hope." The old phrase rang so hollow in his ears he could imagine how it sounded to Merrick.

"Let me take you back to your manager—his name's Norman, isn't it? I'll make the arrangements with him. Here's your hat and cloak."

The Elephant Man trailed Treves down the stairs. In the busy lobby nurses, students, and doctors paused to greet the surgeon and to stare wonderingly at the masked figure with him. Outside, a porter hailed a cab for the pair and they rattled up Turner Street to the Whitechapel Road.

In the shop some coins traveled from the surgeon's pocket to the showman's. Seeing as how it was in the interests of science as well as of his dear friend Merrick, said Mr. Norman, he would cheerfully pilot him to the meeting of the Pathological Society on the appointed evening. As for the Elephant Man, by now he seemed to have sorted things out in his mind. When Treves held out his hand, Merrick shook it long and hard.

On the evening of December 2nd, a group of leading physicians, surgeons, and scientists gathered in the walnut-paneled headquarters of London's Pathological Society. They listened thoughtfully as Treves told the story of the Elephant Man and his strange affliction.

"And now, gentlemen," said Treves, "allow me to present the Elephant Man himself."

Tom Norman was seated at the back of the hall, fondling the silver coins on the chains on his vest. He watched as Merrick, wearing only a robe, stepped forward and took up a position at Treves's side. Something, Norman noticed at once, seemed very different about Merrick.

As a rule, when the little man was exhibited, he looked bored and uninterested. He went through his routine like a sleepwalker. Not so this time. This time his eyes darted back and forth, searching the bearded, bespectacled faces that stared at him. He seemed keyed up and excited, as if something terribly important was about to happen.

Treves whispered to him. Twisting out of his robe, Merrick gave it to the surgeon. The Elephant Man was entirely nude. Chilly though the hall was, he didn't appear to mind. Head held high, he stood unashamed in front of the specialists.

By twos and by threes the members of the society came forward, forming a circle around the Elephant Man. In spite of their gray or bald heads, they looked and behaved like children who had just been given a new plaything. Enthusiastically they pulled at Merrick's strange warty skin and felt the lumps of bone on his head. They bent his arms. They prodded the flaps of flesh hanging from his body. They looked into his mouth. He submitted to everything without a murmur, almost as if it gave him pleasure. Then they drifted back to their chairs.

"One further observation needs to be made," said Treves. "Merrick's condition isn't stable. The tissue growths on his body are becoming larger all the time. So are his head and the bony lumps upon it. . . . Now, gentlemen, have you any comments? Have you come across anything like Merrick's case that may help me to help him while there is still time?"

An elderly specialist from Guy's Hospital stood up. Shaking his head, he declared that in fifty years' practice of medicine he'd never run into a patient with as bizarre a collection of symptoms as Merrick's. Others echoed him. In the present state of medical knowledge, all agreed, they couldn't recommend any treatment to help the unfortunate patient.

The meeting came to an end. In the dark street outside, a sharp wind was blowing. Snow had begun to fall. Treves hailed a cab for Norman and the Elephant Man. The three men shook hands under a street lamp.

"I do have a rare 'un, don't I, Doc?" said Norman proudly.

"That you do. But don't think for a moment I've given up on him. Someone somewhere must have encountered a case* like

---

*Someone had. It was a German pathologist, Friedrich von Recklinghausen (1833–1910), who described a case two years before Treves met the Elephant Man. Because of the German's work the condition is sometimes called Von Recklinghausen's disease. The Elephant Man's case was so extreme, however, it is doubtful that the German scientist would have recognized it as related to the case he studied. See the Afterword at the end of this book.

yours, Merrick. You simply can't be one of a kind. Norman, please keep in touch with me. Let me know if there's any significant change."

"I will, guv, I will."

It was a big step up into the carriage. They helped Merrick mount, and Norman climbed in after him. Chin on chest, his face hidden behind his mask, the Elephant Man sat in silence.

The cabby's whip snapped at his horse's flank. At that moment Merrick lifted his head and, turning toward Treves, waved goodbye. The light of the gas lamp caught the flash of his eyes. The surgeon couldn't be sure, but he thought the little man had been weeping. They were great sad eyes. Eyes that seemed to beg him to help.

Indifferent to the freezing wind, Treves stood there looking after the carriage a long time after it had rolled away.

FOUR

A Constable Interrupts

The least that could be said of Frederick Treves, fellow of the Royal College of Surgeons, consulting surgeon at the London Hospital, and lecturer on anatomy at the London's medical college, was that he was a man of his word. In the months that followed his last meeting with the Elephant Man he continued to seek an explanation of Merrick's strange disease. Each time he looked at the Elephant Man's photographs he felt a surge of pity for the little man.

Deciding that he needed more information from Merrick himself, he set out for the shop on the Whitechapel Road.

As Treves drew close, he could see the gaudy painting advertising the exhibition was no longer in the shop window. He tried the door but it was bolted tight. Peering through the grimy glass, he could detect no sign that the shop was occupied.

He felt a tug at his overcoat sleeve. Looking down, he saw the old-beyond-its-years face of the urchin who had helped him the first time he had visited the shop.

"Looking for the Elephant Man, guv?"

"He doesn't seem to be here anymore. Do you have any idea what's become of him?"

"Can't rightly say. Hit was all the bobbies' doin'. They just didn't like the kind of show 'im an' Mr. Norman was puttin' on. They said it was against public . . . public . . . decency. Mr. Norman, 'e said the poor little man 'ad a right to make a livin'—did they want to make 'im go back to Leicester an' live off the parish? But the coppers, they told 'im to button 'is lip. They made the two of 'em move on."

"Where did they go? Do you know?"

"Out of Lunnon, I s'pose. Mr. Norman, 'e said 'e'd 'ave to go someplace like Nottingham or Stratford, where the bobbies don't make such a fuss about a poor little freak."

If the Elephant Man had disappeared from London, he had not disappeared from the surgeon's mind. Treves wrote up the curious case of Joseph Merrick in an article which he called "A Case of Congenital Deformity," and published it in a leading medical journal. He also discussed the case at another meeting of the Pathological Society. Several physicians came forward with examples out of their own experience that reminded them of Merrick. But the information, interesting though it was, provided no clue to treatment. The case of the Elephant Man remained as mystifying as ever.

From time to time Treves heard from medical men in different parts of the country who had seen the Elephant Man on exhibition. He was reported to be in places like Leicester, Northampton, or Nottingham. One doctor said Merrick was traveling with a show called Sam Roper's Fair. Always he seemed to stay very briefly in one place and then move on. The exhibition of his deformed body apparently was too gruesome for even the easygoing police forces of the countryside to put up with. After a while the surgeon heard no more about him.

Month followed month. As Treves could find no solution to the problem of the Elephant Man's disease, the case began to fade from his mind. However, he could never forget the pathetic, misshapen face of the little man altogether. From time to time it would suddenly appear before him. He would find himself looking into the unhappy brown eyes, with their silent appeal for help, and feel the bottomless anguish in them. He would hear for an instant the odd, high-pitched musical voice and the spluttered, barely understandable words. If only he could have done something to help!

It was a warm, sunny morning in June, 1886. The lecture theater of the London Hospital Medical College was overflowing with eager students. Some of those present, as usual, were much too old to be enrolled in any course. Distinguished surgeons and physicians often turned up at Frederick Treves's lectures, drawn by his sharp wit and brilliant insights.

Treves was standing in the center of the platform, all eyes fastened upon him. From the table in front of him he lifted a shining bony object and held it in the air. The audience craned their necks to see it better.

"Can anyone tell me what this specimen is?"

A student rose. "It looks like a small skull, a child's, sir. But there appears to be another skull attached to it. How can that be?"

"Very good. I'll explain. These are the skulls of the famous two-headed boy of Bengal. I borrowed the piece from the museum of the Royal College of Surgeons. It is possibly the most wonderful specimen in a wonderful collection.

"Gentlemen, you will note these two skulls are joined at the crown. The child was born with an extra head attached, upside down, to the top of his own. He was a Siamese twin—but all that existed of the other twin was the head!

"The child must have been a rare sight. Certainly he was to the midwife. So rare, in fact, that no sooner was the baby born than, with a shriek, the frightened midwife flung him into the fire. Another woman pulled out the baby just in time. Later he was placed on exhibition."

A hand in the audience shot up. "Was the attached head alive?"

"It was alive, with its own brain and other organs, and feelings of its own. If the boy drank milk, we are told that the mouth in the twin head filled with saliva . . . Can you imagine the unhappy condition of a child obliged to go about with his brother's head on top of his own? Still, he did just that until . . . Yes?" The last word was addressed to an assistant, who had stepped out upon the lecture platform.

"Sorry to bother you, sir, but there's a constable who wants to speak to you. He says the matter is most urgent."

Treves dismissed the class and went out into the corridor. A policeman was waiting, hat in hand.

"This card, sir—is it yours?"

Treves glanced at the piece of cardboard the constable held out. It was dog-eared and dirty but unmistakably it was one of his calling cards.

"That's my name, all right. Many people have my card. Why do you bring this one here?"

"Sir, there's a very odd sort of chap turned up at the Liverpool Street Station. Seems to have some frightful kind of disease. He doesn't have a penny on him and he can't rightly make himself understood. But he did give us this card of yours. Could you come with me and identify him, sir?"

A very odd sort of chap . . . with a frightful disease. . . . Treves had handled so many cases that fitted such a description, including some lepers. It was impossible to guess who this one might be. Taking his hat, he went with the constable to a waiting carriage.

At Liverpool Street Station he followed the constable into the third-class waiting room. At one side a policeman was standing guard over something on the floor.

"We found him on one of the railroad platforms, sir. He must have just got off a train. There was a crowd around him, plucking at his cloak and his hat and trying to get a look at him. We shooed them off and brought him in here. He just headed for the darkest corner and collapsed. Hope you can tell us who he is, sir."

Treves looked down at the floor and saw what appeared to be a heap of dirty old clothing that some ragpicker might have thrown away. He bent over for a closer look.

The heap of clothing stirred. A pair of brown eyes stared up at him through a slit in a brown flannel mask under a peaked cap. A hand reached weakly toward him.

Treves raised the flannel. It was Merrick, all right, but a more wretched, ailing Merrick than he had seen before. The little man appeared to be on the brink of exhaustion. The surgeon guessed he hadn't eaten for quite a while. He patted Merrick's hand and turned to the policeman.

"Constable, I know this man. He's in very poor shape. Can you call me a cab? I must get him to the London Hospital."

Treves reached down and helped Merrick to his feet. The Elephant Man made not a sound; he was either too weak or too deeply moved at seeing a friendly face. Treves saw his cane on the floor and picked it up. Taking Merrick under the arm, he guided him out to the street.

The little man sank into the seat of the cab at Treves's side. It threaded its way slowly through the heavy traffic of Liverpool Street toward Whitechapel.

Merrick's head fell on his chest. The surgeon, alarmed, raised the mask. Merrick was fast asleep. He didn't wake until the cab jolted to a halt in front of the hospital.

Treves helped the Elephant Man up the steps and into the lobby. The concerned face of Nurse Ireland greeted him there.

"What have you brought us, Mr. Treves?" Instantly she recognized the strange outfit the Elephant Man had been wearing when she had last seen him. Treves had told her something of Merrick's history. Her quick eye took in his wobbly gait and the way the surgeon was supporting him.

"A new admission," she said. "We can't have him in one of the general wards. It might not be appreciated by the other patients. Where shall we put him?"

"What about one of the isolation wards in the attics? Any vacancies up there?"

The isolation wards were little rooms off the attic wards. They were used in emergencies. A patient might be brought in with a fever the doctors couldn't identify, or he might be delirious, or suffering from a fit. It was to the tiny isolation wards in the attics that such cases were taken. Each room had space for only a single bed.

"There's a room in the east wing just become vacant. We'll take him up there."

Nurse Ireland grasped the Elephant Man under the arm on one side. With Treves supporting him on the other, they half-carried, half-led Merrick up the three flights of stairs and to the vacant room. He never uttered a sound.

They brought Merrick to the bed. He sat down upon it and then, still fully clothed, lay back. Eyes open behind the mask, he stared at the ceiling.

Treves drew Nurse Ireland aside. "Nurse," he whispered, "I want you to help me undress him. Try not to be shocked at what you see. I know you've handled a good many cases that have been maimed or disfigured, but I doubt you've ever had one quite like Merrick. Take what you see in your stride. He may be a sight, but you and I know he has feelings—and they've been put to a sore trial today."

Her blond head nodded. The two began to disrobe Merrick. The hat and mask came off and for the first time she saw the Elephant Man's face. The blood left her cheeks but she continued to undress him. Half asleep, he barely seemed aware of her.

"You poor, poor man, you'll need a washdown." She disappeared and returned with a basin of steaming water, soap, and a towel. Around Merrick's neck was a chain with a large locket which she removed and placed on the night table next to the bed. She washed his entire body, giving him what nurses call a bed bath, and toweled him. Treves, watching, was struck by the new inroads the disease had made on the little man since he had seen him last.

Coolly and efficiently, Nurse Ireland pulled a night shirt over Merrick's body. He submitted without a sound, as if he was enjoying the care, like a child being dressed for bed by its mother. Finished, the nurse tucked him in.

"Nurse." Treves was at the door, ready to leave, for he had urgent business elsewhere. "He'll need a bite to eat. Some hot soup and bread should do the trick."

"Right, sir. I've already ordered it."

"Good. I expect he'll sleep a long time after he's eaten. But tell him I'll drop by tomorrow morning. I want to examine him." The door closed softly behind him.

Nurse Ireland looked at the Elephant Man. His eyes were shut but she doubted he was asleep. Curious, she lifted the locket from the night table and snapped it open. Inside she saw a miniature portrait of a lovely young woman in a blue dress. Who could she be? His sweetheart? That was unthinkable. The nurse closed the locket and returned it to its place.

Since his food would be arriving in a few minutes, Nurse Ireland propped Merrick up in the bed with pillows. His eyes were still shut.

His enormous deformed head leaning against the white pillows, the Elephant Man presented an incredible, monstrous image. He reminded her of something she had seen somewhere. What was it? Suddenly she remembered. It was an Indian idol at the British Museum, its face bizarrely hideous.

Just at that moment someone rapped lightly on the door. Before she could rise to open it, it swung open. In the doorway stood a young wardmaid, a tray in her hand.

The girl took a step into the room. Her eyes came to rest on the face of the man in the bed. No one had prepared her for it, nor had she ever seen such a sight.

"My God!" she shrieked.

The tray fell from her hands. The dishes splintered and the pieces scattered across the floor.

Streaking out of the doorway, the girl disappeared faster than a frightened bird.

Merrick, in his weakened state, seemed not to have noticed. Or had he—and, because it had happened so many times before, learned not to see what he could not bear to?

FIVE

Parade of the Elephants

Joseph Carey Merrick was born in central England, in the town of Leicester. Somehow he could never be sure of the year; he supposed it was 1860, but actually it was 1862. About the day he had no doubts. August 5th. It was not the luckiest day of his life. For his unhappy mother, however . . .

Thank God, he sometimes thought, she isn't alive to see what I have become!

His mother had been a country girl. Mary Jane Potterton was her maiden name, and she came from a village outside Leicester. She was the oldest child of a farm laborer.

Mary's father never learned to read or write. But he provided as best he could for his growing family, and Mary was sent to school until she was twelve. She always loved books and reading, and this love she was to pass on to her son. She walked with a limp but otherwise she was completely normal.

As soon as Mary left school she had to go to work. Every year or two another new brother or sister was born and the family had trouble making ends meet. Mary found a job as a servant in the city.

To her parents, at least, it was a great blessing, for she gave them every penny she earned.

The girl's life was no bed of roses. For fourteen hours a day, year in and year out, she washed and scrubbed, polished and pressed, fetched and carried. But she seemed to thrive on hardship and grew into a very pretty young woman. Joseph had a portrait of her, a tiny one—the kind that is called a miniature. It was his most precious possession. He wore it in a locket around his neck.

Working the long hours that she did, Mary had little time to think of romance. But it came to her all the same, in the person of a young cab driver called Joseph Rockley Merrick. She was already in her twenty-fifth year and she welcomed his attentions. When she found she was going to have a baby, she told the young man and he agreed they'd have to get married. He was to be Joseph's father.

The young couple set up housekeeping in humble quarters in Lee Street. Not very long afterward Merrick, dissatisfied with his earnings, gave up cab driving and found a better job as a warehouse-man in a cotton factory.

Only a short way from where the Merricks lived was the Humberstonegate, one of the biggest streets in the old part of Leicester. Every year, in May, a fair was held in that neighborhood. Large numbers of people streamed into town for the fair. Many came to buy and sell horses, sheep, cattle, pigs, and the like, but there was also a pleasure fair. The Humberstonegate was lined with stalls, scores and scores of them, where for a penny or two you could see acrobats, dwarfs or giants, a horse with five legs, a man with three, a lady with a beard, and other strange sights.

One of the pleasure fair's most popular attractions was Boswell & Wombwell's Royal Menagerie. It was probably the biggest traveling animal show in Britain. It had lions and tigers, zebras and giraffes, baboons, and other rarely seen animals.

To Mary Merrick's great misfortune, it also had elephants.

Every day the Royal Menagerie was in Leicester the elephants were marched through the streets at noon. The sidewalks would be packed with people eager to see the giant beasts parade by.

44

Parade of the Elephants

Mary had a good, healthy curiosity, and when she heard the menagerie was in town she went to see the parade of the elephants. She was in the crowd, toward the front of it, at noon one day in May in the year her son would be born.

A great desire to get a better view took hold of the crowd. They began to push and shove like wild beasts. Suddenly poor Mary found herself being flung out into the road. She stumbled and was unable to keep herself from falling to the ground.

She looked up in fright. A giant of an elephant, its trunk in the air and its eyes rolling, towered above her. One gigantic gray foot was raised and about to come crashing down upon her.

She was terrified. But in her terror she still held on to her wits. She realized she had only an instant left to try to save herself and the unborn child she was carrying. Calling on all her strength, she rolled herself out of the path of the beast and over to the side of the road.

In the next second the great foot was set down exactly where her head had been. If she'd remained in the same spot her head would have been crushed like an eggshell.

Some kind people raised her to her feet. She was so unnerved she needed their help to get home. She never recovered fully from that frightful experience. For the rest of her life she relived it again and again in nightmares.

Three months later her baby was born. They named him Joseph Carey Merrick. Joseph for his father, and Carey for William Carey, a famous Baptist minister.

Joseph's mother was delighted when the midwife told her she'd given birth to a son. Her delight didn't last long. A little before the child's second birthday she found a swelling inside his lip. As time went by the swelling became firmer and firmer until it formed a lump of hard flesh. In the next months it grew into the boy's right cheek. Finally it turned the upper lip inside out and began to push out of his mouth.

One day Mary was examining this growth. Her eyes opened wide in astonishment. "It looks like an elephant's trunk!" she cried to her husband. "That elephant! The one that almost trampled me in the Humberstonegate! The boy has his trunk." And she burst into tears.

When Joseph was five, both of his feet began to grow abnormally large. So did his right arm. The top of his head got bigger and hills of bone grew on it. In different parts of his body the skin became thick and lumpy and covered with warts. The color darkened in places, turning brown and purple.

Mary did as much for her son as any mother could have. She took him to doctor after doctor. Each one examined the boy, clucked over her story of her accident with the elephant, and gave her some lotion to rub into the troublesome parts of the child's body. Nothing helped.

Every year Joseph's old symptoms got worse or new ones appeared. His forehead began to swell up, the first sign of the great loaf of bone that was to disfigure it. A bony mound was noticed on the right side of his head. Little by little it became an enormous lump, which made the ear fold over and left him quite deaf on that side.

Some time later he took a nasty fall. His left hip was injured and the joint became diseased. After that the boy found it hard to get around and to take part in games with others his age.

But even without this accident he would still have had to give up playing with other children. He was beginning to look so peculiar that nobody wanted to come near him anymore. When he tried to join in games, all he heard was "Go home, cripple! We don't play with freaks!" Or: "Stay away or we'll give you what for!"

For Joseph it was hard to understand why children who'd been his friends should turn against him.

In the end he had to resign himself to a childhood spent in loneliness. If he had been dependent on his mother before, now he needed her much more.

Poor Mary! Her life was never an easy one. In less than two years she bore her husband two more children—a son, William, and a daughter, Marion. So she now had these two little ones to take care of besides her oldest child, a hopeless cripple.

For Joseph's father those were not bad years. He changed his job and had been promoted, and now he held the post of engine driver. He moved his growing family to a larger and better home. Ambitious for more money, he opened a small haberdashery shop. As if Mary hadn't had her hands full enough, now she had to manage the shop, for her husband was away all day at work. Young Joseph did what he could to help. After he came home from school each afternoon he straightened things out in the shop or took care of his little brother and sister in the back room.

They'd had the shop about a year when his little brother complained of a headache and nausea and was put to bed. He soon became violently ill. A bright red rash flared over his body. His temperature shot upward. The doctor said the boy had scarlet fever. Medicine could do nothing to help. In just a few days poor little William was dead.

The Merricks couldn't have taken it harder. William was a bright, pretty child. With their first son a cripple, they'd pinned most of their hopes on their second, and now suddenly he was gone. Joseph felt the loss as deeply as his parents.

Neighbors and relatives came to pay their respects to the mourning mother and father, and to say goodbye to little William. Joseph was seated near the open coffin. More than one of the callers, looking down at the little body, said, loudly enough for Joseph to hear, "What a pity! Why couldn't the Lord have spared William and taken the cripple instead?"

No one missed William more than Mary did. For days she hardly ate a mouthful of food. She looked like the ghost of the pretty young woman in the painting in Joseph's locket. In time she began to cough. It was a sharp, racking cough that often left her gasping for breath. To hide her misery from the children she always laughed and pretended to be in high spirits.

One day, about two and a half years later, Mary began to run a fever. Soon she was so weak the doctor was sent for. "Pneumonia," he said. Joseph went to call his aunts, who came to nurse her and take care of the children.

Every day Mary sank a little deeper. But no matter how weak she was or how high her fever ran, she always had a loving smile for her son and daughter.

In just a few days Mary drifted off into a deep slumber. Suddenly Joseph noticed his aunts were sobbing.

"What's the matter?" he asked, frightened.

His aunts only sobbed harder.

He pulled himself over to his mother's bedside. "Wake up, Mother!" he cried. "Please, please wake up!" He covered her hand with kisses.

But his poor mother could neither hear him nor feel his kisses and she never woke again.

She was only thirty-six years old. The night she died, and many nights after, the boy cried himself to sleep. He had lost his treasure, the dearest person in the whole world, the only one who truly loved him. He wasn't quite eleven at the time.

SIX

Outcast

Nothing was the same for Joseph after he lost his mother. For his father too everything was different. His great problem was to make some arrangement for the care of his little daughter, Marion, and his lame son. He solved it by breaking up his home and moving with the children into lodgings.

Their landlady was a Mrs. Emma Antill. She was a young woman, a widow, with children of her own. Merrick paid her to take care of Marion and Joseph while he was away at work. For the time being, a relative managed his shop.

Joseph continued to go to school. With his classmates for a long time he'd had to face the same kind of unpleasantness he had with his former playmates. They wanted nothing to do with him—unless it was to mock his clumsiness or his poor speech and to make him the victim of their cruel jokes. In the schoolroom the desks and seats were double ones; each child sat with a partner. Nobody was willing to be Joseph's partner and sit next to him. The schoolmaster had to place him at a desk in the back, where he sat and worked by himself. He was a good scholar, better than most, because after school there was little for him to do but study and read or help Mrs. Antill.

When Joseph reached twelve his father took him out of school, for twelve was the working age. The boy looked forward to this new chapter in his life with some excitement. What kind of work would he get? Would he find friends at work? Most doors, he knew, were shut to a cripple. But somehow he had to find an open one, for a very pressing reason.

He had a new mother. Mrs. Antill had changed her name to Mrs. Merrick. Joseph's father had taken her to wife about a year and a half after his first wife passed away. Devoted to his dead mother, the boy couldn't understand why his father should want to marry again. Was it because it gave his father a home and a housekeeper free of cost, as well as a manager for his haberdashery shop? Joseph couldn't say. What he could say was that he hated being told he had to call his father's new wife "mother."

He knew at once she would never be a mother to him. She had, after all, children of her own—normal, healthy children. Compared to him they were handsome. His stepmother accepted Marion as her own child, but for Joseph she had little use. He was the pariah of the household.

His stepmother made his life a perfect misery. She was always harping on his failings, especially when his father was about. If the boy had a fault she would magnify it; where he had none she would invent one.

Nothing angered her more than to find Joseph up late at night, reading in bed. She'd come down on him screeching like a witch, snatch the book out of his hands, smack him hard, and snuff out the candle. "Worthless boy!" she screamed. "Wasting a good farthing's worth of wax to read an idle book!"

"It's the Bible, mum," he told her.

"Don't you dare talk back to your elders and betters!" And she smacked him hard again.

None of his stepmother's complaints was wasted on his father. The elder Merrick became increasingly cold and gruff toward his son.

Two or three times the new Mrs. Merrick shamed or tormented

Joseph so much he could stand it no longer. He ran or, rather, being lame, limped away from home. The refuge he sought was the house of his father's younger brother, who owned a barbershop. Uncle Charlie was the best friend he had in those days. Charlie listened to his story, comforted him, and said he could stay as long as he wanted. His father must still have had some spark of feeling for him at the time; he came after the boy and persuaded him to return home.

Joseph's handicap made it hard for him to get about, but his stepmother insisted he go to work; money was short, she kept saying, and he was eating her out of house and home. His father made some inquiries and learned they were hiring apprentices at Messrs. Freeman's, Cigar Manufacturers. Off the boy went to apply for a job.

He found Mr. Freeman a kindly, older gentleman. "We often hire crippled people, Joseph," said he. "As long as they have two hands we can teach them to roll tobacco into the shape of a cigar. We'll take you on trial."

In a short while the boy was rolling cigars as well as the experienced men. His master was pleased with his work. As for his stepmother, she took every penny he earned and still wouldn't give him a kind word.

"That boy of yours will never mend his ways," she grumbled to his father. "If he's as clumsy in the shop as he is at home, he'll be out on the street by Michaelmas." Or: "Now that that boy of yours is working he's a bigger eater than ever. He eats up every single penny he brings in."

During Joseph's first year in the tobacco factory things went fairly well for him. Toward the end of the second year, however, there was a change.

Joseph's right arm and hand had never stopped getting bigger and heavier. He began to have trouble rolling the cigars. He now feared that his stepmother's bitter prediction might come true before long; he was getting clumsier and slower and he was afraid he'd get sacked. He pushed himself harder, rolling each cigar with extreme

51

care. Although his cigars looked better, each week the number he finished was smaller. He waited with dread for the day his master would notice it.

That day wasn't long in coming. Joseph was given a warning; he was told that if he didn't make his quota he'd have to leave. Try as he might—and heaven knows he tried—still the hand grew bigger and clumsier and the number of cigars he rolled smaller.

"It's a pity." Mr. Freeman shook his head. "You're really such a good, hard-working boy. But this job is more than you can do now. I'm very sorry but we have to let you go."

The boy's tear-stained face told his stepmother everything. She flew into a rage.

"Oh, I knew it! I knew it!" she cried. "Clumsy ox! I expect now you'd like nothing better than to sit around at home idle all day reading some stupid book and feeling sorry for yourself. But I won't have it! Out you'll go bright and early tomorrow morning and every morning until you find another job!"

So out he went, morning after morning, dragging himself to factories and shops with a sinking heart. Jobs were scarce, even for the able-bodied. For him there were none at all.

Having no money, when he got hungry he came home for something to eat. "You good-for-nothing!" shrieked his stepmother, glaring at him. "You haven't been looking for work. You've been standing on some street corner looking at girls till you decided it was time for lunch. I'll give you lunch, you shiftless idler!"

She gathered up a few greasy, chewed-over scraps of food ready to be thrown out and flung them at him. "There's your lunch. It's more than you deserve."

Every day it was the same story. Soon the boy could no longer bear to go home to be skewered on her sharp tongue. He stayed out as long as he could, until his hungry belly drove him back to face the dragon again.

Joseph's father suddenly realized there was little hope his son would ever find a job.

"I should've thought of it before," said he. "You can work for me, Joe, peddling things from the shop, door to door. I'll go to the town hall tomorrow and get you a peddler's license. Then I'll fill you up a box with cravats, gloves, and the like, and you'll go out and start ringing doorbells. If the customer wants something you don't have with you, you can bring it to them the next day. What d'you say?"

What could he say? Any prospect looked better than dragging himself about Leicester in search of jobs he couldn't get and going hungry on the streets. He nodded.

"All right, then," said his father. "But remember: this is no schoolboy lark. You'll have to sell enough every day to earn your keep. When you're working for me there'll be none of this here idling your mother complains about."

So there he was, ready to start his new career. His father filled a wooden box with a variety of things from his shop. On top he fitted a tray in which the goods most likely to catch a woman's eye were displayed. With this box hanging by a strap from his shoulders, Joseph limped from house to house, visiting a different group of streets every day. If sales were good his father congratulated himself for having thought of the idea. If the boy came close to falling below his quota he got dark looks and harsh words.

Joseph's stepmother continued to abuse him, no matter what. Nothing he did could ever please her. The sandwich she gave him every morning to take for his lunch was two slices of bread—with drippings on them if he was lucky. At dinner he always found less on his plate than he saw on the plates of the rest of the family.

A peddler, to keep his customers, needs to please them. Joseph could please few. Though he tried to make up for his looks by being as agreeable as he could, people had trouble understanding him. And his face! It was becoming so unsightly it distressed him just to look in a mirror.

He started to wonder why people bought from him at all. Some, he could see, made purchases because he had something they needed and it saved them a trip to the shop. Others bought more out of pity. Still others bought nothing but dropped farthings or pennies on his tray. They simply felt sorry for him. Had his father realized this would happen when he sent him out as a peddler?

Many people wouldn't buy from him at all. When he rang their doorbells they looked out of their front windows, saw the scary-faced lame boy at the door, and fled to the back of the house. Some who opened the door took one look at him and turned about without a word, slamming the door in his face.

For some time Joseph had been wondering what would happen when he didn't bring home money enough to meet his father's expectations. One day he found out.

Evening was coming on and he had been trudging about until he felt so tired he could go no farther. Sitting down on a doorstep, he counted his money. It was much less than the minimum his father had set. The boy's stomach was grumbling with hunger.

Did he dare go home with so small a take? He rested awhile, thinking over the situation.

Suddenly he felt so famished that he rose to his feet and rushed into the nearest food shop. He bought some hot eels and pie and gobbled them down. They tasted as delicious as Christmas dinner.

His hunger satisfied, Joseph realized he'd have to make up the money he'd spent, besides earning the sum he was expected to before he returned home. He started out on his route again.

It was dark already. Through their windows he could see people were at dinner. When they came to the door and found an ugly cripple standing there they were furious. "Go away!" cried more than one. "This isn't the time or place to be begging for pennies."

It was not his lucky day. He turned his face homeward, only too well aware of the trouble waiting for him there.

It met him full on. When he told his father of the poor day's business and confessed he'd spent some of the little money he'd taken in, the face of the elder Merrick turned purple.

"You young rascal! You good-for-nothing!" cried he. "You've been asking for it and now you'll get it!" He balled his fists.

The beating Joseph got was worse than any he could remember.

Paralyzed by guilt and fear, he didn't even try to protect himself His father stopped only when his arms were too tired or his hands too bruised to strike again. Joseph lay on the kitchen floor unconscious.

During the night the boy came to his senses. He was lying just where he'd fallen. He hurt all over and he could taste blood on his lips. In the next room he could hear his father and his stepmother snoring.

I can't spend another night under this roof, he told himself. Taking his few belongings, he thrust them in the bottom of his peddler's box. For his father he left a hasty note saying he would pay him for the goods in the box as soon as he was able. Then, placing the box strap over his shoulders, he hurried out.

The rest of the night he spent huddled in a doorway trying to sleep.

When morning came he immediately set about hawking his wares through the town. That night, and the nights that followed, he slept in a doss house. There, for fourpence, he was given a blanket and allowed to stretch out on a hard, flea-infested bed in company with others as unfortunate as himself. Placing his box at the head of the bed, he propped his pillow against it and attached the strap to his body, for thieves were common in such places.

One afternoon Joseph was making his rounds from house to house when he saw a familiar figure rushing toward him, arms outstretched. It was his uncle Charlie.

"Joseph," cried he, "I'm so glad I've found you! I've been looking for you everywhere since I heard what happened at your house the other night. You poor boy! Where have you been sleeping? How have you been living?"

Joseph told him all in a few words. Nothing would satisfy his good-hearted uncle but that the boy should come home with him at once to be fed a decent meal and to enjoy a night's rest in a decent bed. Further, he insisted that from that moment on Joseph should regard his uncle's home as his own. In his situation the boy couldn't refuse an offer so sincere and generous.

In this way Joseph became a member of his uncle's household.

Each day he would go out and peddle his wares until he was tired, and then return to the apartment over the barbershop. Uncle Charlie treated him like a child of his own, or almost. He didn't require the boy to sell any set amount, as his father had, but just to do the best he could. Every week, for food and lodging, Joseph gave his uncle as much as he could spare, after setting aside some money to pay back his father and some to purchase new goods.

Joseph's aunt treated him kindly. She was a little woman with a good heart and a pretty face. Often he would see a look of sadness pass over it like a cloud. Aunt Jane had brought four children into the world but three of them had died when they were little more than babies. Perhaps she hoped her nephew would take their place.

He hoped so too.

Joseph's disorder continued to grow worse. His aunt did her best to help him to keep clean and control the odor that came from the flaps of flesh hanging from his body but he could see she found it no pleasant task.

It became harder for the boy to get about with his heavy box of goods and to find customers. When he pulled himself from one house to the next, idlers would gather and follow him, gaping. Sometimes children with nothing better to do would run after him and shout insults or pelt him with stones. He could never outrun them. Several times a constable had to come to his rescue.

For two years or so this was the life he led. He felt that honestly he couldn't complain. He had found peace in his uncle's house. He enjoyed a friendliness and warmth he hadn't known since his mother died. Then two things happened that changed his life forever.

The time came when his peddler's license expired and he had to renew it. He made his way to the town hall and applied to the clerk in charge.

The man looked up from his ledger. "So you're the Merrick boy," said he.

"Yes, sir."

"Want to renew your license, do you?"

"Yes, sir, I do."

"There's a problem."

"Sir?"

"We've had police reports about you. And some of the people in town don't like you coming to their homes to sell. Say they find it upsetting. Can't blame 'em, now that I see you. It's against the law to license anyone who creates a public nuisance. I'm sorry, believe me, but I can't renew your license."

Joseph was so shocked he stood there speechless. Slowly he turned around and headed home.

His world had just fallen apart. What was he to do now? How could he earn anything to help pay for his keep? He felt completely lost.

"Don't worry," said his uncle. "We'll manage somehow, lad. Something will turn up."

But nothing did.

Before long Aunt Jane announced she was expecting another child. At the same time Uncle Charlie's business had fallen off and he often complained about it. With the prospect that she'd soon have another mouth to feed, Aunt Jane, Joseph thought, had begun to seem less friendly toward him. He brooded over that.

Finally he told his uncle he felt they could no longer afford to keep him and he didn't want to be a burden to them.

"It's true, Joseph," said Uncle Charlie. "The times are hard and they're likely to get worse before they get better. I've been worrying about you and your future." His sorrowful brown eyes searched the lad's face. He shook his head.

"I can't go back to my father."

"I know better than to suggest it."

"The workhouse.* That's the only place that might have me."

Uncle Charlie nodded sadly. "I wish there was someplace else. I

---

*The English workhouse was a poorhouse where the unemployed, the old, the sick, orphans, and others in need were supported at public expense. The able-bodied among them were compelled to work. Because society assumed that poverty was caused in part by an unwillingness to work, the living provided was often poorer than that of the poorest workman.

hate to see any kin of mine go to the workhouse." He took Joseph in his arms and the boy felt his uncle's tears fall on his face.

They waited until after Christmas. Then Joseph said goodbye to his uncle and aunt and with a small package of his possessions under his arm made his way to the workhouse admissions office. He told the official in charge, a hard-faced man with a frosty manner, that he was homeless and, for reasons that were obvious, couldn't find work.

"Can't find work, eh?" The official shook his head. "They all say that. For reasons that are obvious? They don't all say that. You could do some kind of work, boy, but I suppose your looks are against you."

He filled out the admittance papers. "Don't worry, you won't be idle in the workhouse. Never." He smiled a cold smile. "We'll find work for you. More than you can do."

He was right.

SEVEN

Leicester Workhouse

L eicester Workhouse stood on a height at the city's southern edge, a cluster of forbidding red brick buildings. With every step Joseph took toward the high iron gate his heart sank lower. He showed his admittance papers to the gatekeeper, who waved him to the office.

Inside it felt almost as cold as the raw December day outside. A sour-faced clerk seated on a high stool at a desk greeted the boy with a scowl. He took Joseph's papers, frowned at them, and wrote something in a ledger. "Any valuables?" he barked.

"Only this." Joseph held out two pennies his uncle had given him as a parting gift.

"All money must be surrendered for the support of inmates," the clerk grumbled. "Give them two pennies here." He snatched them from the newcomer and then searched him to make sure that was all he had. "Go to the clothing office. First door on the right."

In the clothing office Joseph was received by another sour-faced clerk, who sat behind a counter. In back of him were shelves piled high with clothing. He took the boy's measurements with his chilly eyes. "Small," said he. "Very small."

Joseph felt himself shrinking as the clerk said it.

Going over to a pile of shabby clothing, the man selected a shirt, jacket, and trousers, then took some underwear and smaller items from other piles. "Carry these into the bathroom over there. Take a hot bath and see you scrub yourself clean. I don't doubt you can use it. Then put these clothes on and bring back the ones you're wearing. We keep them here and return them to you when you leave." He looked at the youth disparagingly. "If you leave."

Obediently Joseph went into the bathroom. It was a big white-washed room with, in one corner, a stove that was much too small for the space it was supposed to heat. An elderly attendant, dressed in a drab uniform like the one Joseph had been issued, stood by the bathtub.

"Here's your hot bath, lad," he said with a smile as friendly as it was toothless. A look of concern took its place when Joseph undressed and the man saw his naked body. He helped the boy into the tub.

The water couldn't have been colder.

"Is th-th-this a hot bath?" asked Joseph, reaching for the coarse yellow soap.

"That's what they call it. But 'tain't hot to me, son, and 'tain't hot to you, so out you come as fast as you can." He held a towel ready for the boy.

Even after Joseph had put on his workhouse clothing (which was rough and gray and reminded him of nothing so much as a prisoner's uniform) he couldn't stop shivering. The bathroom attendant came out with him, carrying his old garments for him, and deposited them on the counter.

"Go with old Bill," grunted the clerk to Joseph. "He'll see you settled in. Now hop to it."

Still trembling, Joseph followed Bill out of doors. The old man had a limp, so he couldn't move very fast, and the boy immediately felt a kinship to him. Bill led him to another building and along endless passageways, each of which felt colder than the one before, and up long flights of stone steps. Finally he stopped in front of a door and opened it. "Here's where you bunk, son," said he.

They entered a room the size of a barracks. Beds lined the walls and more beds stood in rows between them, all very close together. There must have been a hundred of them. Each was covered with a dingy-looking gray blanket and had a tiny pillow.

Bill stopped by one of the beds. "This 'un's yours, son." He pressed a fist down hard on it. The mattress didn't yield a fraction of an inch. "Not the softest you ever slept on, I expect. But beggars, you know . . . Well, you'll get used to it." He opened a small locker. "This is for you. Put your things in here."

Bill stood by as Joseph arranged his clothing, a few books, and other small belongings he'd brought with him. Since old Bill seemed so friendly Joseph showed him the picture of his mother he wore in the locket around his neck and told him about her.

"Sorry you lost your mum so early. It's a pity." He scratched the side of his nose. "But there's a blessing in everything. At least she don't know where her boy is today."

Bill led Joseph downstairs and outside to a big shed. The boy looked about. The place was divided into stalls, each one furnished with a small rude bench and table. Men were seated at them picking over what looked like piles of hemp.

"This here's the workshed," said Bill. "And that big bloke yonder is the workshed master, Mr. Quigger. Mind you do as he says. God help you if you don't. Good luck, son." He limped off.

Quigger was a large man with a mean look and small suspicious eyes. "What, another cripple!" He threw up his hands. "How do they expect me to get any work out if all they send me is cripples and old bags of bones?"

"I'll do the best I can, Mr. Quigger."

"See that you do, boy. We have a lot of rules here. It's me that makes 'em. It's you that don't dare break 'em. If you do—if you break just one—you go to bed without supper. Break it again and you spend a day in the cooler. Shirk your work and it's off you go to the magistrate. Next stop: prison. Have you ever been in prison, boy?"

"No, sir, and never hope to be."

"Good. Good. See that you obey the rules, boy." With a curt nod he led Joseph to an empty stall and set him to work.

So began Joseph's career as a picker of oakum. Every morning a pile of chunks of old hemp rope was deposited on his worktable. These he had to hammer and untwist and pick apart until all that remained were loose fibers. The workhouse sold the fibers to shipbuilders, who tarred them and drove them into the seams between the planks of ships to make them watertight.

Some of those picking oakum were old people. It really wasn't very hard work. But it was for Joseph, who had just one good hand. Quigger set him a quota, four pounds a day. To fill it, the boy's one hand had to do the work of two. If he fell short of his four pounds, Quigger would have a fit and make him go to bed without supper.

Joseph had never enjoyed missing his supper. But in the workhouse going without a meal now and then hardly bothered him. Mealtime there was not a joyful occasion. There was a rule of silence. The inmates sat in a vast, drafty hall, rows and rows of them, with long sad faces, and ate without a word. There must have been eight or nine hundred of them. The men sat on one side, the women on the other. Husbands and wives were separated in the workhouse; at mealtimes they could see each other but weren't even allowed to sit together. If they had children, they were taken from their parents and put out in foster homes. Dismal places those were, Joseph heard.

In the dining hall everyone was assigned a place and given a metal dish for food. Food! It was gruel and bread for breakfast every morning. For lunch an almost meatless boiled joint, or sometimes boiled rabbit. With dried beans. The workhouse must have bought a mountain of dried beans, it served them so often. The tea was lukewarm and tasted like dishwater.

Supper—the inmates called it the tea meal—was bread and drippings and tea. Heaven help the person who asked for an extra slice of bread! The tea meal was at four-thirty. By eight everyone was hungry again. It was a long wait till breakfast.

The workhouse didn't exactly spoil its guests. It tried to give them every reason to move out as soon as they could.

As for Joseph, he had an extra discomfort—the prying eyes and the rude jokes of his fellows. They would never leave him in peace. Were they trying to make up for their own misery by making him the butt of their horseplay? He wouldn't have been surprised.

The workhouse was well named. From dawn to dark it was work, work, work. And bells. At five in the morning a bell clanged to wake the inmates. It clanged to announce the start of a meal and the end of one. It clanged to announce the beginning of the working day. It clanged to announce its close. It clanged at night as a warning the gas lights were about to be turned off and the dormitories closed.

After a few weeks of this slavery and starvation the boy made up his mind he had to get away at any cost. He convinced himself if he made a really hard try to find a job he might have some luck. He wrote to his uncle and asked if he could help. Uncle Charlie came the next visitors' day. The instant Joseph saw his kindly, worried face in the visitors' room he burst into tears. Uncle Charlie took him in his arms and the boy poured out his misery to him. His uncle promised to do anything he could to help. It was agreed Joseph would come and stay with his aunt and uncle while he tried to find work.

The workhouse authorities naturally raised no objection to this plan. And so, dressed in his own threadbare old clothes (which had never looked so good to him before), Joseph shook hands with old Bill and said goodbye to Leicester Workhouse, hoping never to see it again.

Uncle Charlie gave the boy a hearty welcome. His aunt, however, could barely spare the time to greet him. During the twelve weeks since he'd left she had given birth, and the new baby claimed all of her attention. Drawing Joseph aside, Uncle Charlie said he had a cousin who was a foreman in a hosiery factory, and he thought they should call on him. He also said he'd spoken to his minister, who had promised to help if he could.

The visit to Uncle Charlie's cousin was a disappointment. His factory was laying off men, not hiring them—and he didn't know but that he and his family might themselves soon be knocking at the door of Leicester Workhouse.

Uncle Charlie then sent Joseph to the minister. That gentleman had known the boy's mother; she had taught in his Sunday School. He said he'd asked several well-connected members of his parish if they would or could help a poor boy. When they learned the boy was less than able-bodied, they declared they could do nothing for him.

"Your only hope, Joseph," said he, "is in God. Your uncle, you must know, is in no position to keep you. With the new baby it would hardly be fair to look to him for aid."

"Sir, do you mean, then—"

He nodded. "For you I see but one path. Return to the workhouse at once. To your young eyes it may not look like paradise, but if I were you I'd thank God I have it to turn to. Without the workhouse the old, the poor, the sick, the orphaned, and those with handicaps like yourself would be starving in our streets."

Joseph had gone to the minister with high hopes. He left him with none at all. The next morning he took leave of his unhappy uncle and climbed back up the rise to the workhouse. As he walked through the gateway he heard the shrill clanging of the bell. He swore he would never rest until he had left that hateful place behind forever.

For poor Joseph every day at Leicester Workhouse was a torment. From early morning, when he tumbled out of bed to face the sneers of his fellow inmates, until late at night, when he fell into bed exhausted, his life was a black hell. All day his hand ached from the weight of the mallet he used to pound the oakum and his fingers stung from untwisting the rough, heavy fibers.

Some consolations he did have. One was the friendship of old Bill. The boy could always take his troubles to him. If he'd been the old man's own son he couldn't have been treated with greater kindness. And on Sundays there was the chapel. Joseph felt drawn more and more to religion. With so little happiness in this world, it was natural for him to turn his thoughts to the next. Sundays too brought time to read—though all he could lay his hands on were old newspapers and books of sermons. He devoured every piece of printed matter that came his way.

Meanwhile his disease was getting worse. The pink lump growing from his upper jaw—his "elephant's trunk"—had been getting longer every month. Toward the end of his second year in the workhouse this tumor projected inches out of his mouth. It became impossible for him to make himself understood. He had endless trouble in eating too. He couldn't chew solid food, and what he was eating often fell out of his mouth. He became thinner and thinner.

Periodically the workhouse inmates were given a medical examination by a visiting doctor. During Joseph's third year—in 1882—the doctor was struck by the enlarged tumor and sent Joseph to Leicester Infirmary. The surgeon there examined him and said he needed an operation. The only help for Joseph would be to cut away the growth.

"The operation," the surgeon explained, "can be dangerous. You run a strong risk of infection, no matter how careful we are. Therefore you may choose not to have the operation. But if you go on as you are you soon won't be able to take any nourishment but liquids. What do you say?"

All Joseph could do was nod.

The following week he was admitted to the infirmary. It was a welcome change from the workhouse, although he hardly dared to think of what lay before him.

The fearsome day arrived. Afterward all Joseph could remember was being placed upon the operating table, seeing the cheerful faces of the surgeon and the nurses over him, and then smelling the sickly sweet odor of chloroform. When he woke up hours later he was in great pain. But the lump of flesh was gone and he also escaped infection, which took many patients' lives in those days. In a few weeks he was back at his table in the workhouse shed.

How did he manage to live through the terrible years that followed? He never rightly knew. But talking to old Bill helped. Joseph often spoke to him about his dream of leaving the workhouse and of the obstacles that barred his way.

"It's not just my bad arm and leg that make it so hard for me to find work," he was saying one day. "Nobody will hire a person with a face like mine."

Bill slapped his forehead. "Son, why didn't I think of it before? So you do have these problems. But look at them another way and they can become advantages. You like to tell me how your mum was frightened by that great big elephant at the Humberstonegate Fair—"

Joseph's skin had begun to tingle.

"You remember all those funny-looking people on show there— that man with the six toes on each foot, the woman who stuck pins through her cheeks—"

"Freaks, you mean."

"We-e-e-ll, son, you could be one if you wanted. There must be a living in it."

Joseph's stomach squirmed. "Put myself on show? Oh, Bill, you don't know what you're saying! When I find people staring at me or talking about me I feel sick to my stomach."

"Right. But what if all those people pay you for the privilege of staring? Their money's as good as any other. It could take you out of the workhouse. And keep you out. Would that make you feel sick to your stomach?"

"No-o-o, Bill. You've given me something to think about."

"Think as long as you please. But I can tell you who could help you get started. Mr. Sam Torr of the Gaiety. That's the big new music hall on Wharf Street. People say he's always looking for novelties."

"I'm just not sure."

"Write to him, son. Tonight. Can't hurt, can it?"

Joseph decided it couldn't.

A few days later he was called to the visitors' room. A smartly dressed, dapper little man with a diamond stickpin in his cravat was waiting to see him.

"Mr. Joseph Merrick? I'm Mr. Sam Torr. Of the Gaiety Palace of

Varieties, Leicester's finest music hall. You wrote me. And here I am."

He jumped up and pranced around Joseph. Screwing up one eye, the little man inspected him the way a jeweler inspects a stone being offered for sale. Joseph turned red to his ears.

"Hmmm . . . Joseph, that's quite a face you have there. Hmmm . . . I can find a place for you."

"You can't!" Joseph exclaimed in disbelief.

"I can. A good place. As a human oddity." He lowered his voice. "What folks call a freak. It's not the easiest life in the world, mind you. You see, people love to look at freaks but most won't pay to see the same one a second time. A freak's novelty wears out. He has to keep moving on. One week here, one week there, that's the ticket. We need to have lots of different places to exhibit you. If we're to do that, we need some other showmen to go in with us. Leave it to me. I know them all. A-L-L. What do you say?"

Joseph was both dazzled and dismayed. "Yes," he stammered.

"Good, good. Now I want you to tell me everything about yourself so I can pass it on to my mates." He threw out his chest like a proud little rooster. "You can count on Mr. Sam Torr, lad." He fingered the rough gray material of Joseph's workhouse jacket. "This week the workhouse—next week Easy Street!"

EIGHT

Easy Street

The following week Torr called on Joseph again.

"It's all set, me lad," said he, his eyes sparkling as bright as the diamond pin in his cravat. "A new star of the music hall and fairground is about to be born."

"Do you mean your friends, the other showmen, have agreed to go in with you?"

"There will be five of us managing you, Joseph. Me you know. Then there's Mr. J. Ellis. He owns The Living, a spanking smart music hall in Nottingham. Then there's Mr. George Hitchcock, a traveling showman. Then there's Mr. Tom Norman, one of the best of the traveling fraternity. And Professor Sam Roper, owner of Sam Roper's Fair, a very fine touring company."

"I can't believe it!"

"Do believe it, dear lad. An unusual human oddity is a showman's dream. Midgets, dwarfs, giants, and tattooed men are a shilling a dozen. But a curiosity like you? You're a rare one, you are. And will do well. Here, take my card. Come and see me the moment you've discharged yourself from here." He put a coin in

Joseph's palm. "Here's something to seal the bargain." After working the young man's hand vigorously up and down like a pump handle, he departed.

Joseph looked at the silver coin in his hand. A crown! He hadn't seen one in so long it took him a moment to recognize it. Sam Torr certainly had confidence in him! He swore the showman should not be disappointed.

As fast as he was able, Joseph went off in search of old Bill to tell him the good news.

Bill was delighted. "Your luck has turned. Oh, Joseph, I *am* happy for you. A human oddity! You'll make your fortune, son. Your fortune!"

"It will be great to get out of this prison uniform and leave this ugly place behind me."

Joseph regretted his words the instant they were out of his mouth. Poor Bill! Crippled and old as he was, he'd be obliged to remain in the workhouse and wear its uniform until he was carried out in a wooden box.

But Bill was too happy about Joseph's good fortune to have noticed. "Oh, aren't you the lucky one!" he crowed over and over. Then his face grew solemn. "A word to the wise, my boy. Save your pennies. Get yourself a nest egg. Be your own master and you'll be nobody's slave. You don't ever want to find yourself back in Leicester Workhouse."

Joseph couldn't have agreed more heartily. He thanked his friend for his sound advice and many kindnesses and declared he'd never forget him.

On Sunday, August 3, 1884, Joseph pulled off his workhouse gray and put on his own clothing. He hadn't worn it in over four years, and he was so thin it hung quite loose upon him. But at least it was his own. His heart beat very fast as he passed through the gateway—free at last.

The young man soon found himself in Sam Torr's office at the Gaiety, where he received a royal welcome. In the next days he was visited by Torr's fellow showmen. All said they were highly pleased with Joseph and promised to do everything they could to make him a hit.

Torr and Ellis prepared Joseph for his first public appearance. They decided he should be billed as "The Great Freak of Nature— The Elephant Man—Half a Man and Half an Elephant." At first he objected. The words brought back too many painful memories of his poor mother. But in the end he had to admit that the public would find it more attractive than anything he could think of. His managers showed him just how he was to walk and talk and exhibit himself to make the strongest impression on an audience.

Now began a round of appearances in music halls and on the fairgrounds of neighboring towns. To his managers' delight and Joseph's astonishment he was an instant success. Somehow the public found him a great curiosity and they seemed genuinely moved by his tragic story.

Joseph became quite attached to his managers. They were always fair to him and showed him every consideration. He shared fifty-fifty in the money he brought in and they paid all his expenses. Sometimes they gave him gifts besides. He saved his money, or most of it. That wasn't just because Bill had advised him to. Actually there was very little he could spend it on besides books. With his handicaps he was unable to go out to theaters and music halls with young ladies or to go shopping for fashionable clothing. Because of his appearance he couldn't even stay in hotels, like other traveling entertainers. Usually he slept in a show wagon or in a room provided by his managers.

In the fall, with the cold weather coming on, Torr decided to send Joseph to London. He was placed in the care of Tom Norman. Norman operated a number of shows in different shops in the capital.

The police, you may recall, closed down Joseph's show in the Whitechapel Road. After that Norman tried him in outlying parts of London. Then he took him back to Leicester. For some months the young man toured with Sam Roper's Fair. Joseph had his own caravan or show wagon, in which he lived and traveled from town to town.

On the fairgrounds the Elephant Man was often bothered by toughs as he hobbled from place to place. To hide him from their cruel attentions Sam Roper bought him the cloak and the hat and mask that he wore when he first came to Frederick Treves's office at the medical college.

Roper had two burly young men who traveled with the fair and put on boxing exhibitions. They became Joseph's friends and kept an eye on him to see that nobody bothered him. They must have pulled him out of a dozen scrapes.

One incident he would never forget. Sam Roper's Fair had just arrived in Northampton and Joseph was going toward his show tent when three toughs began to tag after him. First they made fun of the way he walked. Then they surrounded him. He couldn't move forward or back or to the side; wherever he tried to go they were there before him, cutting him off. One of them pulled off his cap. Another was tugging at his cloak. The third grabbed his stick away.

He looked about in despair. Not a single one of Roper's people was near. With his feeble voice it was hopeless to cry for help.

All at once he saw the brawny figures of Roper's two young men hurrying toward him. As coolly as if they had been swatting gnats they knocked down the toughs and restored Joseph's stolen possessions to him. Then they picked up the troublemakers and threw them out of the fairgrounds like so much rubbish.

When Joseph wasn't picked on by toughs he was bothered by the police. His managers had never expected to run into that kind of trouble. It wasn't that the police were against freak shows as such. They objected to exhibitions of sick or deformed people. "Morbid," they called the show, and they said they received many complaints about it. Joseph's prospects began to lose their bloom.

One day, after he'd been with his managers about two years, an Austrian showman called upon them. He said he was about to set out for Belgium and he'd be glad to take Joseph on tour with him. He was sure he could find many profitable places to exhibit him

71

there and the police wouldn't hound him the way they did in England.

Joseph's managers took counsel. They decided they couldn't do nearly as well for him as the Austrian said he could and they turned over the young man's contract to him.

The Austrian took Joseph to Dover. As they stepped on the ferry for the Continent he filled his lungs with the crisp, cool air of the English Channel. A whole new future seemed to be opening up for him. His new manager told him that if they did well in Belgium he'd take him to France and to other countries. Joseph could hardly wait.

They landed at Ostend in Belgium. From there they moved on to Bruges, Ghent, and other cities, exhibiting in each of them. Joseph's manager soon discovered he'd made a big mistake. The Belgian police liked the show no better than the bobbies had in London and elsewhere. If anything, they were even more severe. When Joseph and the Austrian arrived in a town, they had to register with the authorities. Soon afterward the police dropped in at the hall the Austrian had rented. As often as not, after seeing just part of the show, they closed it down. Frequently the Elephant Man's stay in a place was just a day or two.

Following the advice of old Bill, his friend in Leicester Workhouse, Joseph had been saving his money. By now he had a nest egg of some fifty pounds. It was more money than he'd ever had—as much as a craftsman earned in a year. Because he had so often been abused and manhandled by rowdies, he never carried it about on his person. In England he'd always left it in the care of Sam Roper or his other managers. None of these gentlemen had ever betrayed the confidence he placed in them. It seemed natural, therefore, for him to follow the same practice with his new manager.

He couldn't have made a greater mistake.

For weeks the Austrian had been complaining about their poor success. He looked for ways to save money, and one of the economies he hit on was that they should share the same bedroom at the inns where they stayed.

They came to Brussels, the Belgian capital. After two days the police closed the show. The next morning, when Joseph woke up, he was surprised to discover that his manager's bed hadn't been slept in. He became very uneasy when he saw that not only the Austrian's clothing but all of his baggage was gone. Joseph hobbled downstairs as fast as he could to learn what had become of him.

Fortunately the innkeeper spoke English and was able to understand Joseph.

"Yes, sir, he's gone," said he. "He settled the bill last night and left after you'd turned in. He said you two gentlemen had a disagreement and you decided to go your separate ways."

"A disagreement? Not that I know of. Where did he go?"

"He didn't say."

Now Joseph had good reason to be upset. He could hardly imagine anything much worse happening to himself than being deserted in a foreign country. He had no friends in Brussels. He was lame. He didn't speak the language or understand it either. Worst of all, except for the few francs in his pocket, his manager had stolen every penny he had in the world.

Joseph climbed back up to his room, sat down on his bed, and tried to think. How could he get back to England? And if he managed to raise the money for his passage, what new misery awaited him when he arrived there? To whom could he turn for help in Britain? Not to his old managers, for they'd made it clear enough they could no longer exhibit him. To his uncle?

Overwhelmed by his misfortunes, he sat motionless, the tears streaming down his face.

After a while self-pity moved out and common sense moved in. First things first, said he to himself. What do you have that can be turned into money—money enough to pay your passage home?

He took inventory of his belongings. Item, the locket with his mother's picture. He could never part with that. Item, a silver watch and chain, a gift from Mr. Norman. Item, a pair of silver cuff links, a gift from Mr. Roper. Item, some new shirts and other linens. Item, a fairly new suitcase. Taking these things downstairs, he

showed them to the innkeeper and asked where he might sell or
pawn them. The man wrote down on a piece of paper the names
and addresses of a few pawnshops and wished him luck.

Carrying his possessions in the suitcase, he went out into the
street. He showed the paper to people passing by and some were
kind enough to point in the direction he had to go. Before long he
arrived at the first of the shops.

Joseph had never been a very forward person. Desperation,
however, gave him courage. Somehow, with the help of sign
language, he was able to make himself understood and to sell his
belongings. The money he received wasn't much—but it would be
enough to get him to the coast, to Antwerp, and to pay for a ticket
there to take him across the Channel and on to London.

As if he didn't have devils enough inside torturing him, he kept
running into others on the outside. Wherever he went he was
hounded by street urchins who wanted to lift up his cloak or his
mask, to pinch him or kick him. When he finally reached Antwerp
harbor, they followed him to the shipping office and right on up the
ferry gangplank.

On the deck of the ferry a sailor blocked their way and chased
them off. Joseph thanked him. But the sailor blocked his way too.

"You're an odd-looking chap," said the sailor. "You'll have to
speak to Captain afore I can let you stay aboard."

When the captain arrived, he told Joseph to take off his hat and
mask.

"What is this loathsome disease you have?" he roared. "Leprosy.
It must be leprosy. You can't cross over to England on my vessel—
my passengers might be infected. Go ashore at once."

Glad at least that the captain hadn't called the authorities, Joseph
hobbled back to the dock. Another ferry wasn't due until next
evening. Buying a bun—his first food in more than twenty-four
hours—he sat down and munched it in the chill and the damp. His
ticket had cost him fifteen shillings, the bun a penny. He hadn't a
farthing left.

The following day, when the next ferry arrived, fortunately no one raised any objection to him. The crossing took all night and it was a rough one. He crouched in a dark, deserted corner to escape the notice of the other passengers.

Very early the next morning the ferry docked in Harwich. Joseph was dizzy from hunger and exhaustion. On the boat train to London he stood in the corridor all the way. He didn't dare enter a compartment and face the stares of his fellow travelers.

He had one hope, and one hope only, when the train pulled into Liverpool Street Station and he climbed down from it.

In Brussels, when he had gone through his suitcase in search of things to sell, he had discovered Frederick Treves's card. The card the surgeon had given him when they met two years earlier. Since then Joseph had been on the point of throwing it away a few times. But somehow he never had.

Now he knew why.

Inside his pocket he clutched it tightly in his good hand, that battered little piece of cardboard.

In all of London, Treves was the only person he felt he could turn to. If the card did not bring him to the surgeon, he was lost.

NINE

The Letter

M r. F.C. Carr Gomm looked angrily over the gold frame of his spectacles. His shoulders seemed to sag. Perhaps that was because, as chairman of the management committee of the vast London Hospital, he carried a very heavy burden. Although the hospital kept growing and growing, it was never big enough. Why, in just the past twelve months alone an unbelievable number of patients—76,000, if the truth were told—had passed through its doors. Extra beds had been crammed into every space available— into corridors and hallways, into cupboards and storerooms—and still there wasn't room enough for all the unfortunates who begged to be admitted.

And now Carr Gomm had just learned that someone who had no right whatever to a bed in his hospital had been occupying one—in a private room—for weeks and weeks. He'd been cared for by Carr Gomm's nursing staff, fed by his kitchens, and treated by his best surgeon—all without the payment of a single penny!

"See here, Treves," he fumed to the young man facing him, "you take too much authority upon yourself." He rapped his metal cigar case on his desk to show how much he meant it. "Don't you know

76

yet that the London is a *general* hospital? It admits only cases in need of active treatment. It does *not* accept people with chronic diseases. It is *not* a home for incurables."

"Quite right, sir." Treves bowed his head contritely.

"Is it not true"—and Carr Gomm gave his desk such a hard rap with the cigar case that a scratch appeared on the polished surface— "is it not true that you admitted one Joseph Merrick, an incurable case, to this hospital? Is that not highly irregular?"

"Most irregular, sir."

"In your report you say Merrick was suffering from exhaustion and undernourishment. Well, now, that might justify keeping him here for a few days or so, until he'd recovered enough to be discharged. But for *all these weeks*?"

"I am at fault, sir," the surgeon replied softly. Carr Gomm's storms, he knew, no matter how they threatened and roared, soon blew themselves out. Each of the two men held the other in the deepest respect. At the same time Carr Gomm, as head of a great hospital, felt he had to maintain a reputation for being firm and evenhanded—especially when he was dealing with Frederick Treves, for whom he had the friendliest of feelings.

Having satisfied his sense of what the world expected of him, Carr Gomm got up and walked to the other side of his desk. Leaning against it, he said confidentially, "Now, Treves, I want to know about this case. It must be a very special one. Tell me—who is this chap Merrick that you should climb so far out on a limb for him?"

"To know who—or what—Merrick is, Mr. Chairman, you'll have to see him for yourself. If you have a spare moment, can you come with me to his ward right now? Good. But before you do, let me tell you his story. He is without a doubt the most moving case I've ever encountered. And you know that here at the London we meet moving cases every day." He opened a large envelope in his lap. "Here are some photographs taken of him when I first examined him a year and a half ago."

"The nurses call him the Elephant Man. Why is that? Does he have elephantiasis?"

"That's what the name suggests, but it's not elephantiasis. Elephantiasis is a disease of the tropics. It's caused by a parasite, a little worm, that may produce swelling in any part of the body. It's spread by mosquitoes. This poor fellow has never been in the tropics. His condition is quite different. It's a case of congenital deformity, and what causes it nobody knows.

"When I first examined Merrick eighteen months ago he was actually enjoying good health in spite of his terrible deformities and a painful hip. Since then he's gone downhill. He's developed a heart condition. And he has a bad case of persistent bronchitis. His disease has also grown much worse. Look at these new photographs I've had taken and compare them with the old ones."

Treves spread out the photographs, old and new, side by side on the desk. Carr Gomm was a hospital administrator, not a medical man. However, even his untrained layman's eye could easily recognize how cruelly the disease had progressed from the earlier set of pictures to the later one. Parts of the Elephant Man's body that looked sound in the first set were covered by ugly skin growths in the second. The lumps of bone on his head were larger. His feet appeared horrendously swollen.

"Poor chap. I've never seen anything so pathetic. How much time do you give him?"

"It's hard to say. A few years at the outside. It's a pity. He used to make a living by exhibiting himself, but he's in no condition to do that anymore. He needs constant care. The only place for him is a hospital."

The young surgeon continued to explain the Elephant Man's case as they climbed the long flights of stairs to the attic. At length Treves stopped in front of a door and turned the knob.

"Merrick, this is Mr. Carr Gomm, our chairman. He'd like to have a few words with you."

Dressed in a hospital nightshirt, Merrick was sitting on his bed, one leg folded under him, the other hanging over the side. In front of him was a large handsome gray structure of cardboard he'd been putting together—a castle, with intricately made towers and turrets, with walls and battlements, with a drawbridge and portcullis. At the sound of the opening door he looked up. The piece of cardboard in his hand dropped to the floor. His twisted jaw fell. His great head shot back and then bent forward. Covering his face, he hunched up his shoulders. He began to shiver as if a blast of cold air had blown into the room.

"Poor Merrick. He can't help it, Mr. Chairman. If someone he doesn't know enters unexpectedly it scares him out of his wits. Come, come, Merrick, there's nothing to fear. Mr. Carr Gomm is only here to make your acquaintance. I promise you'll find him a true friend."

The Elephant Man seemed not to hear. He remained hunched over, his face buried in his hands. A whimpering sound came from his throat.

"Mr. Chairman, he's afraid we're going to throw him out into the street. He has no one to whom he can turn, he tells me, and his greatest fear is that he'll end up in the workhouse. Merrick, the chairman has assured me that will not happen."

"Yes, yes, Merrick," Carr Gomm hastened to add. "It's true the hospital rules won't allow us to keep you here, but I'm confident we can see you comfortably settled somewhere else. I'm going to get off a letter to the Royal Hospital for Incurables this morning. I can't imagine that they won't have a permanent place for you there."

Merrick raised his heavy head and looked at his visitors. His face was wet with tears.

"Honestly," said Carr Gomm, "you need have no fear. You won't be sent to the workhouse. Now tell me—what's this castle you're building here?"

The strange birdlike sounds of the Elephant Man's voice fluttered about the room.

"I'm afraid I don't quite understand," said Carr Gomm.

"Mr. Chairman," said Treves, "I expect I'll have to be his interpreter. I've become used to Merrick's speech and I understand it well. He says he's working on a model of King Arthur's castle at Camelot. Merrick's designed it himself and cut it out of cardboard.

79

He has to work very slowly putting it together—poor chap, he has just one good hand. Sometimes the nurses help."

The Elephant Man's voice fluted again.

"He's almost finished, he says. When he is, he'll feel honored if you'll accept it as a gift."

"Merrick, that's very gracious of you. I should be happy to have it. I know just the place in my office to put it. Thank you very much."

"Please don't thank me," Treves interpreted. "I've read about Good Samaritans like you and Mr. Treves in the newspapers, and honestly I've found the stories hard to believe. But now I do. There really are generous, wonderful people in the world."

"I see you have some books by your bedside," said Carr Gomm, embarrassed.

"I love to read. You understand, I've always had to spend so much time by myself. Books keep me company. Books are my friends—my best friends. Except for Mr. Treves and the nurses, and now you, sir. These are some books he's lent me."

"Very good. Well, I've enjoyed meeting you, Merrick, and I hope you won't mind if I drop in again. Right now I have to get off my letter to the director of the Royal Hospital. I want you to stop worrying. We're going to do our best for you." With a wave and a reassuring smile, Carr Gomm left the room.

Some weeks later Carr Gomm met the surgeon in the lobby of the medical college. "I was just coming to see you, Treves." He held up a letter. "It's about Merrick. From the Royal Hospital for Incurables. You know, we've been corresponding back and forth. I've done my level best, but the upshot is they refuse to take him." Carr Gomm shook his head. "I simply don't understand these people. But they say that even if we paid they wouldn't consider him acceptable. They're afraid the sight of him would be too disturbing for their patients and staff. Can you imagine—*disturbing*—in a hospital for incurables?"

"Bad luck. I don't know how I'll break the news to him."

"For heaven's sake, don't. There's still another place I can try, the

British Home for Incurables. Perhaps they'll have some little room where he can be isolated. By the way, drop in at my office and have a look at Merrick's castle. I'm going to show it to the members of the hospital management committee when they call. We've got to win all the support we can for poor Merrick—just in case."

But after weeks of correspondence the British Home for Incurables declared Merrick just as unwelcome a prospective inmate as the Royal Hospital had.

"We can't go on much longer this way, Treves," Carr Gomm confided. "If I continue to keep Joseph in the hospital I'll be in hot water with my committee. And I can't turn him out either or he'll surely end in the workhouse. And that, I know we both agree, would kill him."

"There must be somewhere else we can turn."

"There is. The English public. Englishmen have good hearts. If they could see Merrick and understand his terrible situation I'm sure they'd help. It's up to me to reach them."

"How will you do it?"

"Through the *Times*. It is the most important newspaper in the country, after all, isn't it? I'm going to write a letter to the editor. If he prints it I think we have a fighting chance."

"More power to you, Mr. Chairman."

"Thanks, Treves. I'll need it." Carr Gomm turned back to his office. Sitting down at his desk, he thought for a moment. Then he dipped his pen in the inkwell and wrote:

"Sir—I am authorized to ask your powerful assistance in bringing to the notice of the public the following most exceptional case. There is now, in a little room off one of our attic wards, a man named Joseph Merrick, aged about twenty-seven, a native of Leicester, so dreadful a sight that he is unable even to come out by daylight to the garden. He has been called 'the Elephant Man' on account of his terrible deformity. I will not shock your readers with any detailed description of his infirmities, but only one arm is available for work."

Carr Gomm paused. He tried to recall what Treves had told him about the Elephant Man. He would need to tell it all, the whole pathetic story, so that the readers of the *Times* would feel for the misfortunes of Merrick as deeply as both Treves and he did.

"Some eighteen months ago," he continued, "Mr. Treves, one of the surgeons of the London Hospital, saw him as he was exhibited in a room off the Whitechapel Road. The poor fellow was then . . . endeavouring to warm himself over a brick which was heated by a lamp. As soon as a sufficient number of pennies had been collected by the manager at the door, poor Merrick . . . exhibited himself in all his deformity."

The chairman's pen flew on, telling how the Elephant Man's exhibition had been stopped by the police. Merrick, unable any longer to earn a living in England, had gone to the Continent with a new manager. "The police kept him moving on, so that his life was a miserable and hunted one." One day his manager disappeared, taking with him Merrick's life savings. He was alone and penniless in a foreign country. But he did have some things he could pawn to get enough money for his passage back to England. He believed that there, if he could locate Frederick Treves, who had befriended him, he might be helped.

Merrick had found Treves, Carr Gomm related. The London Hospital had taken him in and he was "being treated with the greatest kindness—he says he has never before known in his life what quiet and rest were." But the hospital's rules wouldn't let it keep him and both of the hospitals for incurables had refused to accept him.

"Terrible though his appearance is," Carr Gomm continued, "so terrible indeed that women and nervous persons fly in terror from the sight of him . . . yet he is superior in intelligence, can read and write, is quiet, gentle, not to say even refined in his mind. He occupies his time in the hospital by making with his one available hand little cardboard models, which he sends to the matron, doctor, and those who have been kind to him. . . .

"It is a case of singular affliction brought about through no fault of himself; he can but hope for quiet and privacy during a life which Mr. Treves assures me is not likely to be long.

"Can any of your readers suggest to me some fitting place where he can be received? And then I feel sure that, when that is found, charitable people will come forward and enable me to provide him with such accommodation. . . .

"I have never before been authorized to invite public attention to any particular case, so it may well be believed that this case is exceptional. . . .

"I have the honour to be, Sir, yours obediently,

F.C. Carr Gomm, Chairman, London Hospital.

November 30, 1886."

Carr Gomm read over what he had written. "Now, Joseph Merrick," he said, "I've done all I can for you. If this letter is published and it helps people to know you and care for you as we do, your troubles may be over. If it fails . . ."

He continued to read the letter over but the lines on the page began to waver. Shaking his head, he hurriedly addressed the envelope.

TEN

Elephant House

"I can't believe it! I simply can't believe it!"

The Elephant Man had shot bolt upright in his bed, sending the book in his lap flying. Mouth wide open, he stared in disbelief at the surgeon.

"Why should I lie to you? It's true, Merrick, I swear. You aren't headed for the workhouse. The House Committee—you know, the hospital's governing board—held a meeting last week. They've authorized Mr. Carr Gomm to keep you on indefinitely. I've been away with my family, visiting Dorset, and I've just found out myself."

The good left hand rose, palm upward, in protest. "But, Mr. Treves, the London doesn't take in incurables like me. You told me so yourself. So did Mr. Carr Gomm. It's against the rules."

"You're quite right. But sometimes the only human thing to do is to bend the rules. That's what the committee decided to do in your case."

To Merrick the news was too good to be true. It was difficult, if not impossible, for him to grasp that a creature like himself—who had to hide his face behind a mask and slink along deserted alleyways—should be accepted as a permanent inmate by the great London Hospital. All of his experience, his instincts, told him it had to be a cruel hoax.

"But I can't pay, Mr. Treves," he spluttered in his birdlike voice. "Why should the committee let me stay if I can't pay? It makes no sense."

"It makes very good sense. The fact is, you can pay and you will. I showed you Mr. Carr Gomm's letter in the *Times*, didn't I? It's brought dozens and dozens of replies. Lots of them contained money. In just the first week or so he received upward of two hundred pounds, all earmarked for your support. And the letters and money are still pouring in."

"Two hundred pounds! Two hundred pounds . . . from people who don't even know me!" He gestured toward his face. "I suppose if they could see me they'd want their money back."

Merrick, the surgeon saw, would take some convincing. He sat down on the chair next to the bed. "I think just the opposite." He paused for his words to sink in. "But I haven't told you all. The chairman has also received a very generous letter from a gentleman named Singer. He offers the London fifty pounds if it will keep you this year—and fifty pounds next year and every year after that. So I should say we have enough to take care of you in style. Besides, the press is picking up your story all over the kingdom, so now the money's coming in from just about everywhere."

The Elephant Man moved his head from side to side in a wide, emphatic sweep. "Mr. Treves, it all sounds too wonderful. I don't deserve it. Something is bound to happen to spoil it for me. I feel it in my bones. You yourself will leave the London to go to some other hospital. Or Mr. Carr Gomm will. There'll be someone else in charge. He'll decide I'm too horrible to look at and should be put away someplace where no one can see me."

Treves drew his lips together in a solemn line but his eyes twinkled playfully. "I see you refuse to be convinced. Well, tell me—where do you suppose they could put you where no one would see you?"

85

"I've often thought about it. In a lighthouse. Like the Eddystone Light, off the coast at Plymouth. I saw a picture of it once—a lonely column of stone, miles out at sea. Out there no one could suddenly open a door the way they do here and peek in at me. And I could work there! I could take care of the light. That can't be too hard. The only person who'd need to see me would be the boatman, when he came to deliver provisions and oil for the light, and I'd wear my hat and mask then. Wouldn't that be the perfect home for me?" A note of pleading came into his voice, as if he had only to persuade the surgeon and his wish would be granted. "Mr. Treves, I'll work for nothing—just for my keep. I promise I'll never, never leave the lighthouse, not even on holiday!"

"I'm afraid you're letting yourself get carried away, old chap. I know a few lighthouse keepers. They don't live alone—usually there are two or three of them. And they do have to be in good health . . . and able-bodied."

"I see." Merrick brooded a moment. Then his eyes lit up. "What about an asylum for the blind? I've sometimes thought how happy I could be in a home for the blind. No one would see me there, would they? No one would be frightened half to death by me. And—" He stopped abruptly and flushed, as though he'd been about to say something he shouldn't.

"And?"

"Well . . . there might be some blind young woman there . . . some good-hearted blind young woman . . . who might . . . because she couldn't see me as I really am . . . who might take a fancy to me." He tried to turn it into a joke. "You know, they say love is blind."

"I understand." Treves spoke more softly. "But haven't you forgotten something? Asylums for the blind are for the *blind*. They do have firm rules about not accepting as an inmate a person like yourself, who can see."

"Oh! I don't know much about the world, do I?"

"You're learning. It may interest you to know that among the letters Mr. Carr Gomm received were some recommending a lighthouse and an asylum for the blind as shelters for you. He didn't take them very seriously. One letter was even more extreme."

"What did it say?"

"That we should seek to place you in Dartmoor Prison. You know, that dismal place on the moors in Devonshire. The worst criminals are locked up there, each in a cell by himself."

"All by himself? All by himself?" He seemed to relish the words. "I shouldn't mind that at all, I think, even if it is a prison. I could read all the day long in my cell or learn to make baskets. Do you suppose—?"

"I suppose it might be possible, Merrick—if you robbed a bank, wrecked a railroad train, or did something else of that sort. But somehow I don't believe you have it in you. And, speaking of a cell of your own, you'll soon have to give up the one you're occupying."

"I don't understand."

"This room. It's an isolation ward, actually. The hospital needs it for emergency cases. Besides, you're much too well-to-do a gentleman to remain in cramped quarters like these. We have grander plans for you. You're to have a little apartment of your own. Downstairs."

Merrick's eyes shot wide open. "An apartment of my own? Where is it? Can I see it?"

"It doesn't exist yet, at least in a finished state. We're remodeling the rooms for you. It will be very private—much more private than the cell you wanted in Dartmoor. It could be ready in a couple of weeks."

"Oh?" Merrick's voice trembled with eagerness. "Please, Mr. Treves, can you show me where it is?"

"Why not? Come along. I'll take you there directly."

Raising himself from the bed, Merrick took his hat and cloak from the closet. He put on his enormous slippers and picked up his cane. Treves led him to a back stairway, where they would be less likely to meet someone who might be startled by the Elephant Man.

They reached the lowest level of the hospital, the basement. Ahead of them they heard the sound of hammering.

"Are we nearly there?" asked Merrick breathlessly.

"We are there now." Treves pushed open a door.

On the other side of it, a workman on a ladder was hammering a loose board in place. Buckets of paint were clustered on the floor; next to them lay a tarpaulin. Sawdust and pieces of board were everywhere. In one wall there was a fireplace, on another a window and a door. It wasn't a large room and it was quite disorderly.

"Hallo there!" The workman looked down in surprise at his two visitors. "Mornin', Mr. Treves." His eyes lingered on the Elephant Man and his unusual costume. He smiled. "And you"—he addressed Merrick—"must be the Elephant Man. I saw you once when you was in the Whitechapel Road. It's a pleasure meetin' you 'ere like this, in person."

Merrick, who had been looking around the room, fluted a reply. The workman didn't understand, but that hardly disturbed him. He climbed down from the ladder and said, with the tone of a proud proprietor, "Don't judge this room by 'ow it looks now. It'll be a beauty 'fore I finish. A bedroom–sittin' room, fit for a real toff—I mean a gent. Why don't you come along and let me show you the rest?"

He led Treves and Merrick back into the corridor, where he opened another door. Inside, a grimy plumber, wrench in hand, was tightening a pipe. It was attached to what was unquestionably a bathtub.

"This," said Treves, "will be your bath. You're to have a bath of your own. Like it?"

"A bath of my own?" Merrick almost crowed. "I can't believe it. Imagine! A bath of my own!"

Merrick limped back to the bedroom with Treves. The workman, who followed, took up his hammer again.

"Come here, Merrick." Treves was standing by the narrow window. "Look out there . . . That's Bedstead Square. We call it that because that's where the workmen bring the hospital bedsteads when they're in need of painting or repair." He gestured toward the door near the window. "That's your private entrance. Now that's something I don't think anyone else in the entire hospital has—an entrance of his own. It makes you someone very special."

Merrick said nothing. He had the air of someone lost in a dream. He wasn't standing in an unfinished little room in a hospital basement. He was in the chambers of a gentleman in Mayfair, elegantly furnished, spacious, and airy. He barely heard what Treves was saying.

"You can go in and out as you please. I expect after dark will be most suitable. It will be nice, on a summer evening, to walk about and enjoy the night breeze. And I'll show you how to get to the hospital gardens on the other side. You'll like them."

Merrick recollected himself. "I'm very happy, Mr. Treves. I don't think I've been so happy in all my life. A place of my own! I've never even dared dream of having one. I can't thank you enough. And please, please thank Mr. Carr Gomm and the gentlemen of the committee. I simply can't believe this is happening to me."

The workman had picked up a paintbrush and was swishing paint on the wall. He couldn't resist listening to the conversation or at least the part of it he could understand. Nor could he resist taking part in it. "We're all very 'appy for you, Mr. Merrick. Oh, you're quite a celebrity at the London, you are. Everybody in the 'orspital is talkin' about you. They keep comin' in to see how your quarters are comin' along. They've even made up a name for the apartment. Bet you can't guess what it is."

Merrick looked at him expectantly.

The workman chuckled. "They call it the Elephant 'Ouse."

There was a twitter of sound from the little man. Treves decided he had joined in the chuckle.

The handle of the door turned. Nurse Ireland poked her neatly capped blond head inside. "Ah, Mr. Treves. I've been looking for you everywhere. Mr. Carr Gomm has just received a letter. From Leicester. He thought it was very important. He said you should discuss it with Mr. Merrick at once." Her soft blue eyes smiled at Merrick as she handed Treves the letter and left.

"Let's see what this is all about," said Treves, putting on his glasses. "From Leicester, eh? That's where you're from, Merrick, isn't it?"

The Elephant Man made no reply. His eyes rested on the floor. Treves, busy reading the letter, failed to see his face had gone white.

The surgeon cleared his throat. "This letter is from a man who signs himself Charles Merrick."

Merrick looked up. "Uncle Charlie!" He was trembling.

"He's read about you in the papers. He invites you to come and live with him and his family. He says you can stay as long as you want."

"Uncle Charlie!" A shadow passed over Merrick's face. He took a deep breath. "I knew it! I knew it!" he cried. "I knew I wouldn't be able to stay here. I'll have to go to live with Uncle Charlie now, won't I?"

"That depends. How do you feel about it?"

"I feel . . ." Tears were running down his cheeks. "I lived with Uncle Charlie once before. He was good to me—better than my own father. But he has children. And a wife. I was another mouth to feed. And not a very handsome one at that. Do you have any idea how happy his family will be to see *me* again?"

Treves nodded. "I think I do. Want my professional opinion? The hospital is the only proper place for you. You do need special care, and you're likely to need more and more as time goes by. I doubt that your aunt and uncle can provide it. And besides—"

"Besides?"

"Besides, what should we do with all the checks and pound notes that keep pouring in to the hospital? We'd have to return every single one of them—and we don't have the slightest idea where half of them came from. No, Merrick, I'm sorry. The best and the easiest thing for all concerned is to keep you here. Provided—"

The Elephant Man held his breath.

"Provided, of course, that you agree."

ELEVEN

A Lady Comes Calling

M ens sana in corpore sano," murmured Frederick Treves to
himself. "A sound mind in a sound body."

Like every true surgeon, Treves was more than a mender of
diseased or broken bodies. He regarded himself as a healer of the
whole man. Now that he had provided for Joseph Merrick's physical
well-being so far as he could, he felt he must look to his patient's
mental health.

Treves had often seen the frightened look that came over Joseph's
face when the door of his room was accidentally thrown open by
some thoughtless porter or wardmaid. One day when he was visiting
Joseph a wardmaid had pushed the door open to allow some of her
friends to get a peek at the hospital's greatest curiosity. He would not
soon forget how Joseph had cringed and hunched up his shoulders
in fear—and how, after Treves had threatened the woman with
dismissal, Joseph had pleaded for her with tears in his eyes.

The Elephant Man needed and wanted the friendship of his
fellow humans but he was afraid of them. In his mind he was the
most hideous creature on earth. He was a thing so vile, he believed,
that people were right to shun and abuse him. Nor, Treves felt,

would he ever think better of himself until he found that people could value him in spite of his handicaps.

In his basement apartment Joseph was cut off from the busy world of the hospital. He saw few people. The house surgeons came to his rooms every day (Treves had ordered them to) and so did some wardmaids and nurses. But, except for Treves, Nurse Ireland, and one or two others, they came only because their duties called them there. They examined Joseph or helped him bathe or cleaned his rooms and then got out as fast as they could.

Most of these visits, Treves saw, were so routine and impersonal they only served to remind the little man how different he was from his visitors. They made him feel all the more that he wasn't a human being like the rest. He must meet more people—especially people from outside the hospital—and learn that they could care for him for his own sake.

The Elephant Man's apartment had been made as cheerful and attractive as possible. It was furnished with a comfortable armchair, a table and chairs, a bed, and other pieces, including a bookcase that held Joseph's growing library. A vase of flowers brightened the mantelpiece. Colorful pictures decorated the walls. One thing the apartment did not have—a mirror. The surgeon believed if Joseph were not reminded of how he looked he would in time become less self-conscious.

If Joseph were to have visitors and feel comfortable with them he couldn't receive them in a hospital robe or the clothing in which he'd arrived at the London. Calling on his tailor, Treves asked him to come to the hospital and take Joseph's measurements. A jacket and shirts were created for him with one arm larger than the other, and special trousers. A pair of leather shoes was ordered from an orthopedic shoemaker.

On Treves's next Sunday visit—he tried to look in on Joseph once a day and to spend two hours with him every Sunday—his patient greeted him in his new outfit. The little man limped proudly back and forth across the room.

"I feel like a king," said Joseph. "I know I don't look like one. But how do you like my new suit?" He turned around.

"Upon my word, it's really wonderful. I must compliment my tailor."

"I owe it all to you, Mr. Treves."

"Oh no. The money wasn't from me but from the funds given for your support."

"I do wish there was a mirror in the room so I could see how I look."

"No mirror? Well, you can believe me, you look fine. Where did you get that rose on your lapel?"

"Nurse Ireland brought it. She *is* sweet."

Carr Gomm's letter in the *Times* and the newspaper articles about the plight of the Elephant Man had aroused much interest in him. Sympathetic people applied to the hospital to visit him. Treves made sure he or one of his surgeons was present whenever any of them called.

None of the visitors, however, were ladies. And it was precisely ladies, in Treves's opinion, that Joseph needed to meet. Women were more horrified by him than men, and their mindless panic when they saw him always stung him sharply. If he could meet a woman who would look at him with friendly eyes instead of frightened ones he might begin to see himself not as a monster but as a man.

"The situation," observed Treves to Carr Gomm one day, "calls for delicate handling. I plan to invite a young woman—one that is friendly, attractive, and well dressed—to the hospital and introduce her to Joseph. I'll ask her to greet him, shake hands, and chat with him for a few minutes. That should be enough for a start."

"Do you have any particular young woman in mind?"

"I know a number who meet the requirements. But who among them can come face to face with poor Merrick and play her part without getting upset?"

"What about an actress? Theatrical people are used to disguising their feelings. Do you know an actress?"

"I know Madge Kendal. Now there's a real actress—and she's also a charitable lady, ready to help out in a good cause."

"Splendid! You must go and apply to her at once."

Madge Kendal was at home when Treves called.

"The Elephant Man!" she exclaimed. "Of course I know of him. I saw Mr. Carr Gomm's letter in the *Times*. In fact I sent some money to help and persuaded my friends to do the same. My husband has been to see him and was deeply touched. He said Merrick has the most musical voice."

"Then you will come?"

"I only wish I could. But with the play I'm appearing in and the new one I'm rehearsing I don't see how I can. Perhaps there's something else I could do?"

"The poor chap needs more things to fill his time. He passes so many hours alone in his room. Even a leper isn't so isolated—he's with others of his own kind."

"I know just the thing! A gramophone. He can have a wonderful time listening to cylinders of music on it. I'll send some along with the machine. I suppose he's up to winding it."

"It's a grand idea. I'm sure it will make him very happy." The surgeon rose to go.

"Wait just a moment." Mrs. Kendal opened a drawer, took a photograph out of it, and began to write on it. "I can't come to visit your patient in person yet. But I can in a photograph." She held it out to Treves. "I hope he likes it."

Treves gazed at the picture of the great actress, handsome, round-cheeked, and smiling, just as she looked at that moment in front of him. Across the bottom she had written: "For Joseph Merrick—with warmest good wishes. Your friend, Madge Kendal."

"An autographed picture of the Queen of the London Stage! Merrick will treasure it. Thank you very much."

During the following weeks the surgeon asked several other ladies to visit his patient. All were interested but hesitant. One day an attractive young woman friend was calling on him and his wife. Her name was Leila Maturin and she was the widow of another surgeon. Treves put his proposal to her.

"I've told you what he looks like. The visit may be a trying one—but it will all be over in a few minutes. For this gentle, unfortunate man it will mean more than you can imagine. It will tell him he isn't as horrible as he's persuaded himself. And it will help break down the wall of fear that shuts him away from other people."

"Freddie, you have a good heart. I do want to meet your Merrick. Can we go tomorrow?"

The next afternoon Treves led the young widow down to the basement of the London Hospital.

"Merrick, this is my friend Mrs. Maturin. I've told her all about you and she's eager to make your acquaintance."

Joseph struggled to his feet, flushing. He looked at the smiling young woman. If only he could think of something to say!

With an easy grace Mrs. Maturin took in both her hands the left hand hanging limp at his side. She shook it. "I'm so pleased to meet you, Mr. Merrick. I've brought you a book by Jane Austen. Mr. Treves tells me you're a great reader, and I know you'll love it. Would you mind very much if I write to you from time to time?"

Joseph took the book without a word. Then he sat or rather sagged down into his armchair. A great sob came from his throat. Bending his enormous head forward, he buried his face on his knees. Treves had never heard sobs so deep and long.

The interview was at an end.

Next day Treves looked in on Joseph.

"Please apologize for me to Mrs. Maturin," begged the little man. "I hope you can forgive me too. I shouldn't have broken down like that. But I couldn't help it. Aside from the nurses, Mrs. Maturin is the first woman who's smiled at me in years." Tears welled up in his eyes. "And I think she's the first woman that ever offered to shake hands with me. The first woman in my whole life."

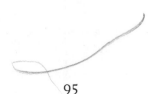

CERTIFIED COPY OF AN ENTRY OF BIRTH

GIVEN AT THE GENERAL REGISTER OFFICE,
SOMERSET HOUSE, LONDON.

The statutory fee for this certificate is 3s. 9d. Where a search is necessary to find the entry, a search fee is payable in addition.

Application Number 90038

REGISTRATION DISTRICT Leicester

1862 BIRTH in the Sub-district of East Leicester   in the County of Leicester

Columns :—	1	2	3	4	5	6	7	8	9	10
No.	When and where born	Name, if any	Sex	Name, and surname of father	Name, surname, and maiden surname of mother	Occupation of father	Signature, description, and residence of informant	When registered	Signature of registrar	Name entered after registration
395	Fifth August 1862 43 Lee Street Leicester	Joseph	Boy	Joseph Rockley Merrick	Mary Jane Merrick formerly Potterton	Warehouseman	M. J. Merrick Warehouse 43 Lee Street Leicester	Twentyninth August 1862	Machentro Registrar	—

CERTIFIED to be a true copy of an entry in the certified copy of a Register of Births in the District above mentioned.
Given at the GENERAL REGISTER OFFICE, SOMERSET HOUSE, LONDON, under the Seal of the said Office, the 29th day of October 1964.

This certificate is issued in pursuance of the Births and Deaths Registration Act, 1953. Section 34 provides that any certified copy of an entry purporting to be sealed or stamped with the seal of the General Register Office shall be received as evidence of the birth or death to which it relates without any further or other proof of the entry, and no certified copy purporting to be given in the said Office shall be of any force or effect unless it is sealed or stamped as aforesaid.
CAUTION.—Any person who (1) falsifies any of the particulars on this certificate, or (2) uses a falsified certificate as true, knowing it to be false, is liable to prosecution.

*See note overleaf.

BX 105062

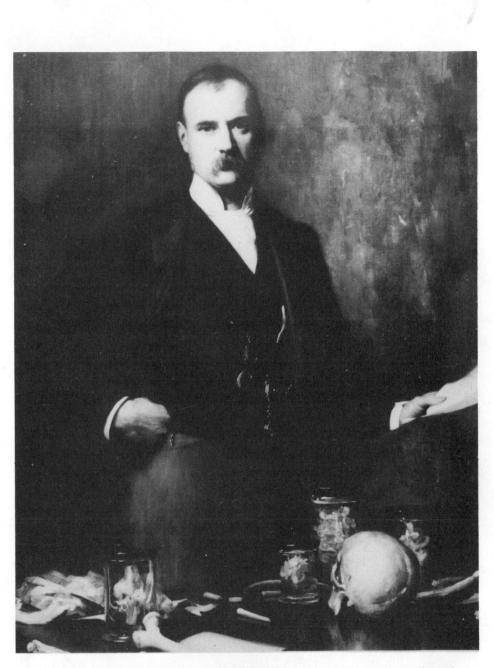

Portrait of Sir Frederick Treves by Luke Fildes, which hangs in the Medical College of the London Hospital.

Copy of the registration of Joseph Merrick's birth.

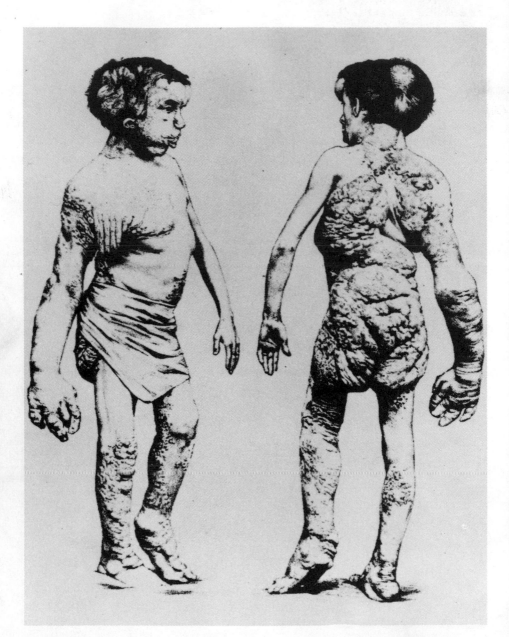

Joseph Merrick as he appeared when Frederick Treves first examined him in 1884. Note the delicate left arm and the overgrown right one. (*Transactions of the Pathological Society of London*, vol. 36, 1885).

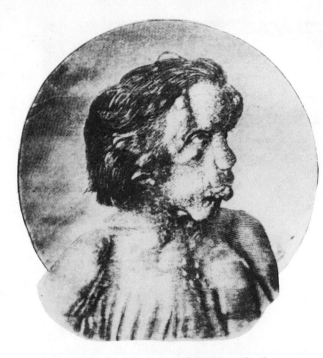

Joseph Merrick as he appeared in 1886, after he was admitted to the London Hospital (*British Medical Journal*, December 1886).

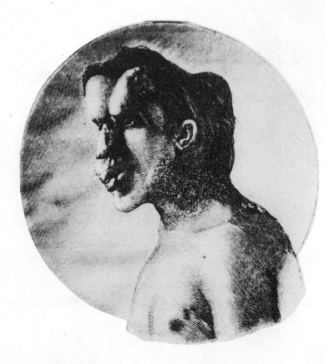

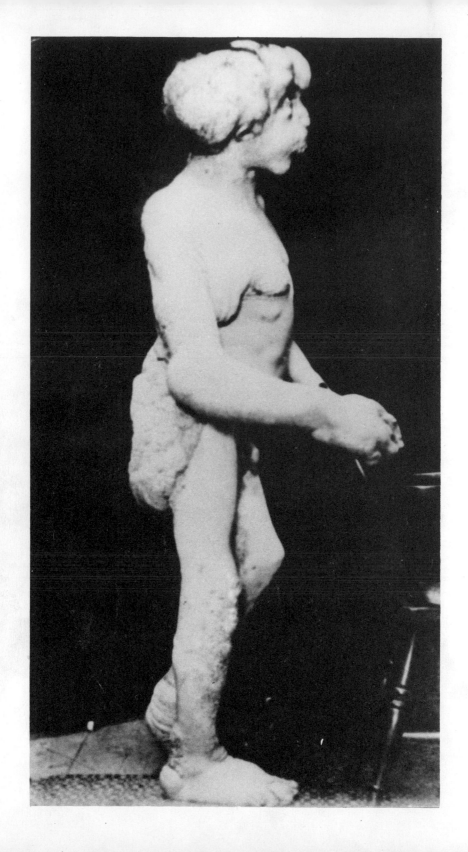

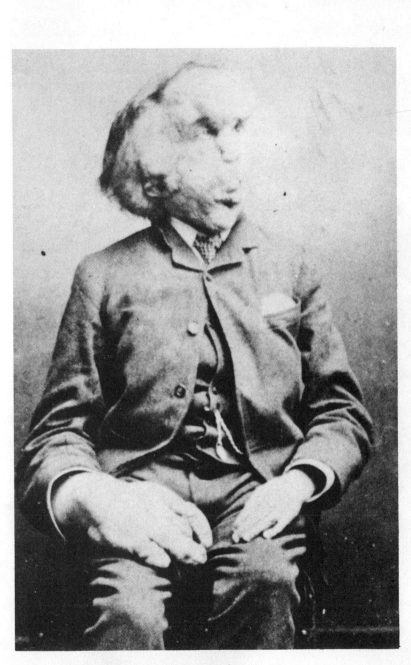

Joseph Merrick poses for his photograph.

Opposite: Photograph of Joseph Merrick taken at the time of his admission to the London Hospital in 1886.

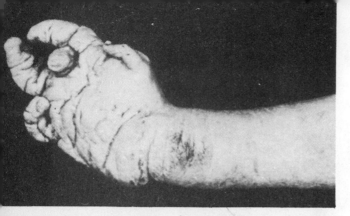

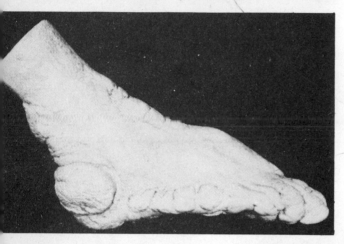

Casts of Merrick's right arm
and hand (showing the palm)
and his right foot, made after
his death.

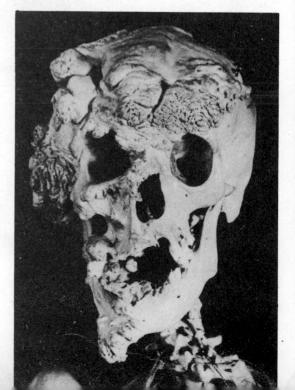

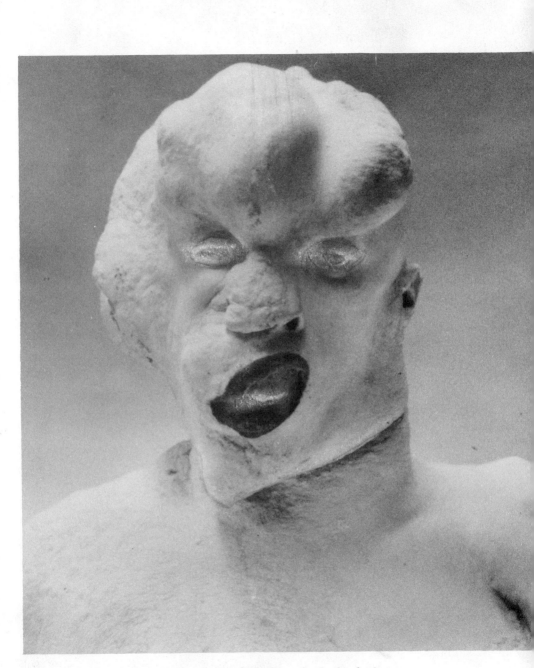

Cast of Joseph Merrick's head, made after his death.

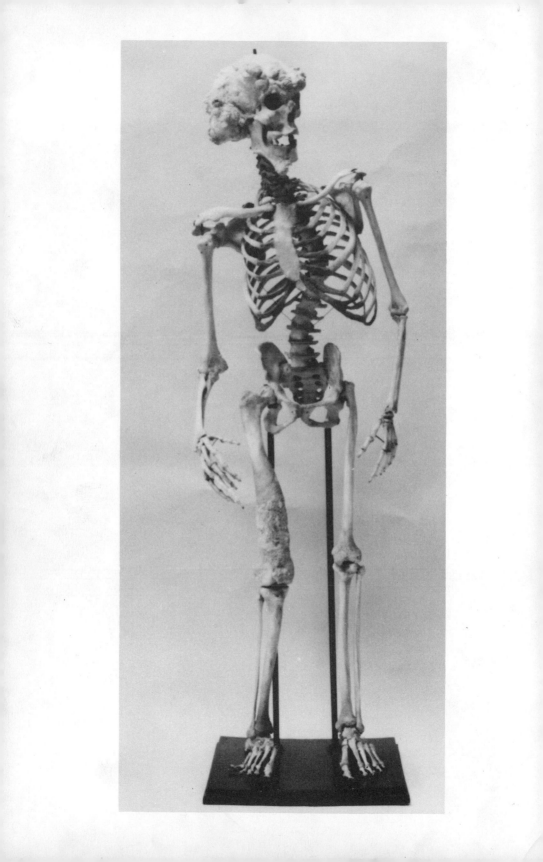

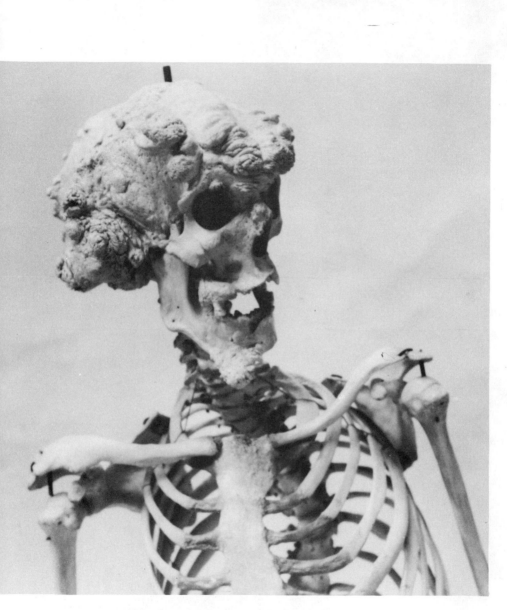

Joseph Merrick's skeleton, showing the deformed skull, curved spine, diseased left hip joint and overgrown right thigh bone.

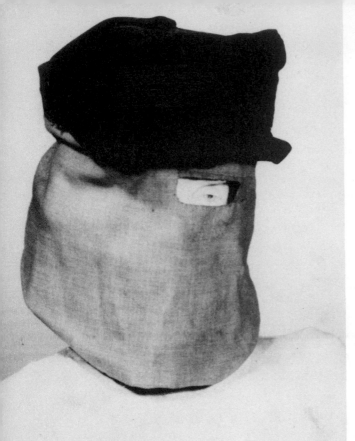

Top: The Elephant Man's hat and mask, still preserved at the London Hospital.

Bottom: The entrance to Merrick's rooms off Bedstead Square at the London Hospital, as it appears today.

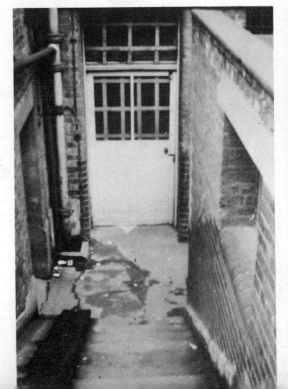

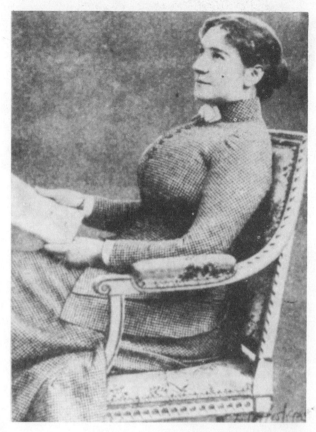

Top: The actress Madge Kendal, one of the Elephant Man's early patrons (*Herald Tribune*).

Bottom: Cardboard model of a church made by Merrick as a gift for Madge Kendal.

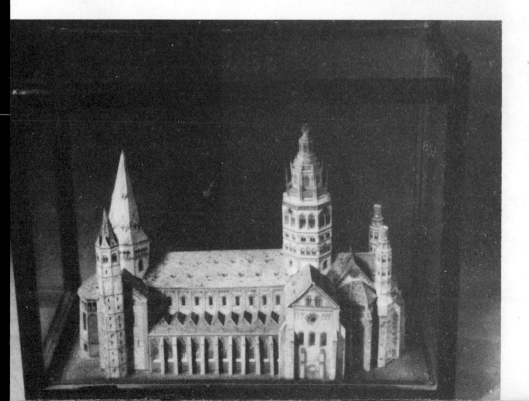

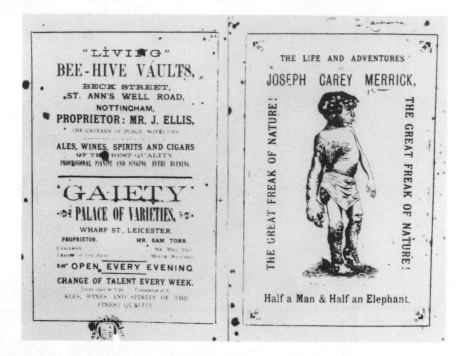

The back and front covers of Joseph Merrick's brief biography, sold at his performances (British Library).

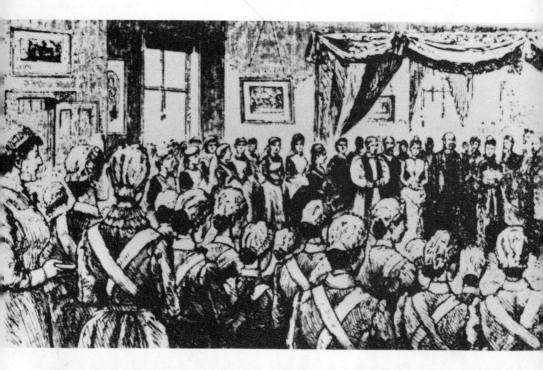

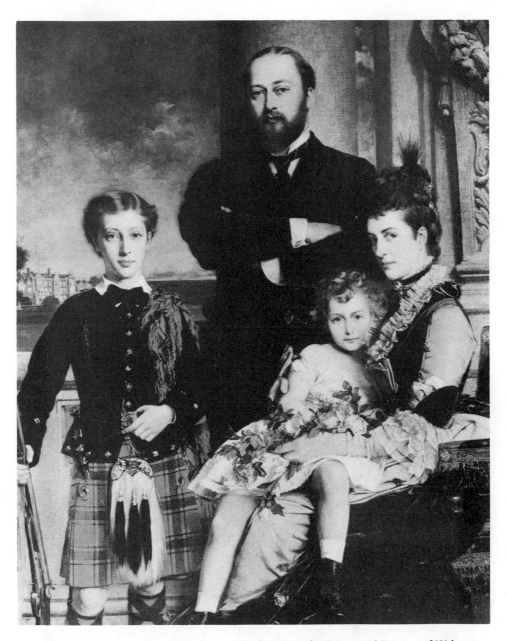

The Elephant Man's two most distinguished visitors, the Prince and Princess of Wales, with two of their children (painted by Von Angeli, 1876).

Opposite: Alexandra, Princess of Wales, opens the London Hospital's new Nurses Home on May 21, 1887. Shortly afterward, she visited Merrick in his basement apartment.

TWELVE

Fit for a King

Bright spring sunlight spilled through the basement window and the glass panels of the door. It struck the polished frames of the photographs on the mantelpiece and set them sparkling. It fell on the face of a porcelain shepherdess and warmed her dreamy smile.

"I love my little apartment," said Joseph to Treves, who was visiting him that Sunday morning. He gestured toward the mantelpiece. "The gifts from my visitors make it look so wonderful. Did I tell you this is the first real home I've had since I was a child?" His delicate left hand moved up and down on the arm of his chair, keeping time to some tune he'd heard on his gramophone. "Of course it can't be nearly as grand as your house in Wimpole Street."

"Grand? My house? My house isn't grand at all. It's really quite small. And with my two daughters getting bigger, and patients overflowing from my waiting room, why, it feels smaller every day."

"But it must be so much bigger and more elegant than any house I've ever been in. I'd give anything if I could see what a *real* house looks like inside. Not one like the little houses I grew up in in Leicester. No, a *real* house. I mean a house with a hall . . . a

96

drawing room where guests are received . . . with old family portraits on the walls . . . a staircase . . . and a big dining room with a real sideboard and a great silver punch bowl and tea service."

"Well, as I said, my home is quite small. But it does have some of the things you mention." Images flashed through Treves's mind of the cramped homes the Elephant Man must have known—of drafty, dingy lodging houses, of sideshow wagons, of the grim workhouse. A visit outside would fit in perfectly with the surgeon's plan for broadening his patient's narrow world. "Would you like to pay a visit to my house? It could be a pleasant change from the hospital."

"A pleasant change? Why, sir, it would be one of the most exciting moments of my life!"

Treves smiled at his enthusiasm. "Then we'll go there very soon. How would next Sunday suit you? I'll pick you up at eleven and take you home with me. Mrs. Treves and the girls have heard so much about you I know they'll be delighted to meet you in person."

"Oh no! Do you really think they will?"

Punctually at eleven the following Sunday the door to the Elephant Man's apartment opened. Treves found his patient dressed in his new outfit, impatient to go.

Twisting out of his armchair, Joseph straightened his clothing. "Do I look all right? I do so want to make a good impression on Mrs. Treves and the young ladies."

"Young ladies? They're just little girls—one's four, the other eight. But I'm sure you'll make a fine impression."

The cab dropped them in front of Treves's house. They made a curious pair, standing side by side on the pavement, the tall surgeon in his top hat and frock coat and the little Elephant Man in his peaked cap and mask and long black cloak.

Joseph looked at the trim little building in disbelief. "Is this really 6 Wimpole Street, sir?"

"Well, it's not Buckingham Palace." The surgeon pointed toward the shining brass knocker on the door. "Why don't you announce our arrival the way any other guest would?"

A maid opened and curtseyed. Treves had prepared her and the rest of his household for the appearance of the Elephant Man.

"Give your hat and cloak to Mary, old chap," he said. "Please feel at ease. There's nothing to fear. You're simply going to meet some new friends, like the ones you've been meeting at the hospital."

Mrs. Treves and her two daughters, Hetty and Enid, were waiting in the drawing room. At the sight of the surgeon's wife Joseph stiffened up. Then he saw the children and his self-consciousness melted away. Uttering a birdlike sound of delight, he bowed. The girls, their eyes so big they looked as if they would pop out of their heads, curtseyed and shook Joseph's hand. They wished him a pleasant visit. They would have liked to say more—much more—but their mother marched them firmly off to the nursery.

Joseph, supporting himself with his stick, watched as the three went up the staircase. Even after they had disappeared he stood there waiting, as if he hoped they would return. "Your daughters are adorable," he said. "Mrs. Treves is so lovely. She reminds me of my mother. I must tell you about my mother sometime."

"Yes, I'd like you to." Treves took him gently by the arm. "Let's begin our tour."

Slowly the surgeon showed his guest from chamber to chamber. Joseph couldn't move very fast; his bad hip was hurting and, besides, everything he saw stirred a childlike wonder in him. He stopped to touch the drapes, to sit in an easy chair, to inspect the lamps, to examine the paintings on the wall. He counted the straight-backed chairs arranged in neat rows in the waiting room and the corridors.

Coming to a mirror, the Elephant Man paused and stared at himself.

Quickly Treves took his arm. "Here's something I want to show you." He turned a doorknob. "This is my consulting room. Would you like to step inside?"

Joseph studied the titles of the medical books on the shelves. He inspected the desk, the anatomy charts on the wall, the medical instruments.

Somehow the surgeon felt his visitor wasn't as impressed as he had expected to be. "It *is* a small room—perhaps the smallest consulting room in all London," said Treves, almost in apology.

"And to think that in this little room you receive duchesses and dukes and millionaires." Joseph clucked in astonishment. "It's hardly larger than my own room at the hospital. . . . I am feeling tired now, Mr. Treves. Can I say goodbye to your family?"

On the drive back to the London Joseph seemed unusually silent and thoughtful.

"I can see," said Treves with a chuckle, "that your visit was something of a disappointment. You were prepared for a magnificent house, like one of the great mansions you've read about in those romantic novels you're so fond of. You expected to see footmen scurrying about in powdered wigs and livery, and maids who spoke French, but there were none. The staircase was just plain old English oak instead of fancy imported white Italian marble. Why, there wasn't a single gilded mirror in the whole place, was there?"

"I was surprised, if you don't mind my saying so. I had expected something quite different."

"Didn't I warn you my house isn't very grand?"

"Oh, Mr. Treves, sir, please don't think I was disappointed. Far from it. I was just surprised at first that someone so famous and important as you should have so small a house. But when I thought about it, I realized it was just what I should have expected. You are, sir, if you'll forgive me for being so personal, a practical man. You are direct and modest. Your house is just like you. That's only natural, isn't it? But . . ." He paused, as if uncertain whether he should continue.

"But what? Go on, man."

"But your beautiful wife and those two lovely little girls of yours!" He closed his eyes and sighed. "They are fit for a king!"

THIRTEEN

Excitement in Whitechapel

With shaking fingers the little man straightened the silver chain that hung across his vest. (Like the silver watch to which it was attached, it was the gift of a generous duke.) His suit had been pressed, and his shoes had been polished till they shone like glass. His apartment had been scrubbed and dusted till it was spotless.

Anyone else would have been satisfied. But not Joseph. Not on this day, May 21, 1887.

Heaving himself out of his armchair, he hobbled across the room to the mantelpiece. He shifted a curio a little to the left. He straightened a painting on the wall. Then he moved the curio back to where it had been.

At last, settling in his chair, he rehearsed his speech. It was a short one, as speeches go, no more than a handful of words. He'd been over it a dozen times and he was sure he knew it by heart. But when he tried to run through it the thirteenth time he couldn't remember how it began.

Almost despairing, he looked at his watch. Thank God! He still had an hour or two to go over the speech and get it letter-perfect.

The door opened. His old fear of strangers started him trembling.

But it wasn't a stranger. Nurse Ireland beamed at him and her smile was like sunshine, calming and warming. He would have smiled back but he couldn't, any more than he could show any other expression. He could weep but he could not smile.

"Joseph, you should see the sidewalks on Whitechapel Road! You wouldn't believe how packed they are. Why, the whole East End must be in front of the hospital, hoping to get a look. It shouldn't be long now. I'll be back to keep you posted." She waved and disappeared.

The whole East End! Joseph could understand their eagerness. He was, if possible, more eager than anybody.

After all, it wasn't every day you got to see the Prince and Princess of Wales.

The Prince and Princess of Wales!

The London had been home to Joseph for almost a year now and he loved it. Still, it was a hospital and most of his time he spent by himself. But this was one day when it was exciting to be a patient there. He wouldn't have to stand outside for hours in the jostling crowds. He wouldn't have to stretch his neck to catch a glimpse of the royal pair. The Prince and Princess were coming inside. They were coming to dedicate some new hospital buildings. And, incidentally, they were going to visit several of the wards.

One patient, and one patient only, had been selected to be visited privately by the Prince and the Princess.

For any Englishman, noble or commoner, a personal visit from his country's future King and Queen would have been a very special honor. For a poor unfortunate like Joseph Merrick it had to be a glory indescribable. Small wonder, then, that he hadn't slept all night and had been waiting anxiously all day for their coming.

Just thinking of it made him dizzy.

A half hour ticked by. Or was it an hour? Joseph couldn't be sure. Then Nurse Ireland was back, out of breath, standing in his doorway.

"They arrived exactly on time," she said. "The Prince is certainly as handsome as his pictures. The Princess has just declared the new nurses' home open. Now the royal party's going through the

101

children's ward. What a warmhearted lady the Princess is! I could see the tears shining in her eyes when she talked to the sick children."

"Nurse, you don't think she'll cry when she visits me, do you?" Joseph blinked nervously.

"I should think not! I've never seen you looking so well, Joseph. And in that handsome Bond Street suit of yours. Oh, no, you are quite admirable." And, patting him on the shoulder, she left.

To Joseph it seemed like a hundred years before Nurse Ireland returned. Her cheeks were flushed and her blue eyes sparkled with excitement.

"They're coming! They're on their way down the staircase now. They'll be here any moment." She bent over and straightened his tie. "I hope you'll mind your manners."

"I hope so too. But honestly I don't know what I'll do, I'm so nervous."

"Joseph, I'm sure you'll make us all proud of you." She vanished.

A minute or two later the door swung open and Frederick Treves stepped in, smiling. Joseph had never seen him so splendidly dressed. Even Treves, always so firm and calm, looked a trifle insecure. He'd just been telling the Prince and Princess what the Elephant Man looked like—but he never could be sure how people would react when they came face to face with him for the first time.

The royal party swept into the room. Joseph, dazed, found himself on his feet, bowing. He knew he was supposed to say something, but what was it? He couldn't remember a word.

"Please be seated, Mr. Merrick," said Princess Alexandra with a gracious smile.

A chair was placed for the Princess next to Joseph's armchair.

"I am so pleased to see you, Mr. Merrick. We've read and heard so much about you. Mr. Treves tells me that, with your patience and sweet temper, you are an example to us all. Here, I've brought you some flowers."

Joseph took the bouquet and stammered his thanks. The Princess talked to him while Prince Edward, stroking his whiskers, examined the photographs on the mantelpiece with interest.

"Hallo! Whom have we here? Why it's Madge Kendal." He winked. "You have some handsome lady friends, Mr. Merrick."

Joseph, crimson with embarrassment, nodded his great head.

Princess Alexandra gestured toward the table. "Who made that lovely basket?"

"I did, Your Highness. I love to weave baskets."

The Princess couldn't understand Joseph's strange speech. She looked puzzled. Treves explained what he'd said and the Princess smiled.

"How long have you been weaving baskets?"

"I've just begun. Thanks to Mrs. Kendal. She has sent me a teacher. God bless her, she is a good-hearted lady."

"And a wonderful actress too," said the Princess, standing up. "We must go now, Mr. Merrick. The Prince still has to dedicate the medical college building. Please, there's no need to rise." She shook Joseph's hand. "I enjoyed our little visit. I hope I may call on you again and stay longer the next time I come to the hospital."

Overcome with awe and gratitude, the little Elephant Man could only bow.

A few days later a package addressed to Joseph arrived at the hospital. Treves brought it down at once.

"It's something special," said the surgeon. "You'll never guess who sent it."

Joseph unwrapped the gift as fast as he was able. His eyes filled with tears.

"What is it?"

Mutely Joseph passed it to him. The surgeon found himself looking at a photograph of the Princess of Wales. At the bottom she had written, "With kindest regards. Alexandra."

Taking the photograph from Treves as if he feared the surgeon might damage it if he held it too long, Joseph carried it to the mantelpiece. He moved some pictures away from the center and placed the photograph there. Then, facing it, he bowed.

He was still standing there, gazing at the picture as if in a trance, when Treves stepped softly out of the room.

Later Joseph also received a gift from the Prince of Wales, some grouse he himself had shot on his country estate. The little man penned letters of thanks. He showed them to Treves.

"Should I change anything?" he asked anxiously. "Is it correct to begin a letter with 'My dear Prince' and 'My dear Princess'?"

Treves read the letters over. The spelling was good but the letters didn't have the proper language, the courtly phrasing that etiquette called for in addressing royalty. However, every word glowed with the adoration of a man who was worshipful and sincere.

"I wouldn't change a comma, Merrick. I don't think anyone at the royal court could write a better letter."

News of the visit of the Prince and Princess of Wales to the Elephant Man spread from the court through the highest social circles in England. It wasn't long before some of the noblest and wealthiest people in Britain were paying visits to Treves's patient. Joseph, for so long the most despised and rejected of men, was suddenly a social success.

Day by day, Treves noticed, the little man was less alarmed when his door opened. He looked less haunted, less anxious, less eager to hide. He seemed to feel at ease not just with wardmaids and nurses but with elegant ladies, with dukes, with generals, with leaders in many professions who came to call. Yet he never lost his gentle, sweet nature or his appreciation for the kindness he was shown.

At the London a circle of friends had begun to form around Joseph. Sometimes when the surgeon came in he found his patient at the window chatting with one of the workmen outside. He'd become acquainted with many of the people who worked around Bedstead Square and enjoyed talking to them. He loved to show the hospital staff the presents he'd received from his patrons, and he always expressed amazement that he should be so favored. One employee's son, who was studying violin, would bring his fiddle to Joseph's apartment in the evening and play for him, and then the two would listen to his gramophone, which was a great novelty in those times.

He is changing, mused the surgeon, just as I hoped he would. He no longer thinks of himself as a freak, a monster more hideous than

Victor Hugo's hunchback of Notre Dame. In part that is because there are no mirrors about to remind him how unsightly he is. But also it must be because he's found that people don't turn away from him once they've really come to know him. His goodness and sweetness, like a powerful light, shine through so brightly, people barely see his deformity.

And, because they care for him, at last he can care for himself.

FOURTEEN

The Kiss

F rederick Treves bent over before the fireplace in the Elephant Man's basement apartment. He stirred the coals until the flames shot sparkling up the chimney.

It was a Sunday morning in December, 1887. Other medical men, their weekday cares behind them, might choose to sleep away a cold winter Sunday morning. But not Surgeon Treves. Every Sunday morning he came early to the London to visit each of his patients and to find out how they were progressing. Treves knew that Joseph especially hungered for company. He had other visitors, of course, but most of his day—week after week, month after month— he had to spend in his tiny apartment, solitary as a monk in his cell.

"What's the weather like outside?" asked the little man.

"Why don't you go to the window and see for yourself, lazy-bones?" Treves, an athlete, a sailor, and a long-distance bicyclist, was a firm believer in the value of exercise. He knew that poor Joseph got hardly any and, with his bad hip, could do very little at best. The surgeon always encouraged him to move about as much as possible in his apartment, especially in winter, when the weather was often too unpleasant for him to venture out on the hospital grounds.

The Kiss

Joseph raised himself from his armchair. Cane in hand, he limped over to the narrow window and raised the blind. Outside he saw a world of white; a freezing fog filled Bedstead Square.

"Christmas is almost here," said Treves significantly.

"It will be a very good Christmas for me." Joseph glanced around his snug chamber. With its pleasant furnishings and books, its mantelpiece and table covered with vases of flowers, photographs of elegant ladies, pretty knicknacks, and curios, it looked more like the apartment of a matinee idol than a hospital shut-in. "I never dreamed I'd have such a handsome little home of my own. Why, I feel like a real gentleman."

"Yesterday I was out shopping for gifts for my daughters and my wife," Treves continued. "The girls had such a list of things they wanted! Tell me . . . is there something special *you'd* like for Christmas?"

"Well . . . I'd dearly love to go to the theater. Would you believe it, Mr. Treves—I've never been to the theater in my whole life?"

To Treves the revelation hardly came as a surprise. It took little imagination to picture what might happen in a theater if the Elephant Man, in his long black cloak and great hat, were suddenly to appear in the doorway. Every eye would follow him as he went lurching down the aisle. When the curtain rose the drama would take place not on the stage but wherever he was sitting.

"By George," declared the surgeon, "that's a situation that should be remedied. Come to think of it, it's high time you had an outing from the hospital. A visit to the theater—what a capital idea!"

"Yes, but . . . how could I go? There'd be such an uproar in the theater. Why, once in Nottingham I tried—" He hunched up his shoulders at the recollection.

Treves's cool hand touched his wrist. "Don't worry, my boy. I think we can work this one out. By the by, do you know that Christmas is pantomime time in the theater? How'd you like to see a pantomime?"

"Very much. What's a pantomime?"

"It's a play and yet it's more than a play—it's a spectacle. It's a drama, a comedy, a music hall, a ballet, all in one. It has actors, singers, dancers, clowns, make-believe animals, an orchestra. It has troops of gorgeous girls too, and scenery so fantastic it will take your breath away. All the parents in London who can afford it take their children to see the pantomime at Christmas time."

"Nobody ever took me. . . . Yes, I'd love to see the pantomime."

"Let's see what we can arrange. Our friend Mrs. Kendal knows just about everyone in the theater. I'll get in touch with her at once. I expect she can pull a string or two to help us."

The notion of a trip to the theater captivated Joseph. "What theater shall we go to? What will the pantomime be about?"

"The Drury Lane Theatre's putting on *Puss in Boots*. Do you know the story?"

"Mmm. I think I do. My mother read it to me when I was little. I'd love to see *Puss in Boots*. Please, Mr. Treves, can you arrange it?"

"We'll see what we can do. Tell me, is there anything else you'd especially like?"

A faraway look came into the Elephant Man's eyes. "Well-l-l, there is something." He riffled through some papers on his table and picked one up. Shyly he held it out to the surgeon.

Treves read the piece of paper. It was an advertisement clipped from a newspaper. "Gentleman's Dressing Case," it said. "Complete with everything the man-about-town needs: silver-backed brushes and comb, ivory-handled razor, toothbrush, silver shoehorn, ciga-rette case, and hat brush."

A gentleman's dressing case? Certainly an odd choice for some-one like poor Joseph, thought Treves. Dressing cases are for travel-ing, but he's not going anywhere. The rest of his days will be spent in the hospital. Marveling at Joseph's request, the surgeon read the advertisement over again.

Silver-backed brushes and comb. Poor Joseph would have a devil of a time straightening his hair with them. Every month it became thinner and more scraggly as the weird outgrowths of flesh and bone got bigger and uglier, taking over more of his scalp.

An ivory-handled razor. Even less useful, because the skin that covered his face was so abnormal it was unnecessary to shave.

A toothbrush. An ordinary toothbrush would be of little use to him—his mouth was too malformed to work the brush across his teeth.

An ordinary hat brush would hardly be suited for brushing his odd peaked hat. And he already had a shoehorn to get his feet into his orthopedic shoes. The cigarette case? Joseph didn't smoke. Even if he wanted to, he couldn't manage it; his lips could not hold a cigarette.

All at once the surgeon understood. As he'd observed dozens of times, Joseph, although a grown man, was in many ways still a child. Like any child he loved make-believe. Treves's little daughters enjoyed putting on their mother's shoes and hats and pretending they were grown-ups. A string of beads and a gilt cardboard crown could transform them into princesses or queens. In the same way Joseph, looking at his dressing case in the privacy of his apartment, could imagine he was a suave young man-about-town, a Don Juan, going off to spend a weekend at some mansion in the country where he would meet and enchant half a dozen lovely young ladies.

Joseph already had a few such gentlemanly possessions, which he treasured. A nobleman had given him a stylish mahogany walking stick with a knob of silver. From a lady he'd received a gold ring, which he wore proudly on one of the fingers of his good hand. But no gentleman's silk hat could ever fit on his great dome of a head. His giant misshapen feet could never fit into a gentleman's pair of patent leather shoes. The suit that Treves's tailor had made for him was presentable enough, but on his deformed body it would never look smart.

But he could at least have a handsome dressing case. And that case, in his imagination, could take the place of all the things he did not have and never could. In the world of make-believe he could be everything he would never be in the real one.

"Well," said Treves with a sympathetic wink, "let me borrow this advertisement. I'll see what can be done."

Christmas was drawing closer and closer. With every mail Joseph received handfuls of colorful cards from gentlefolk and lords and ladies who had visited and befriended him. Each card he greeted with exclamations of astonishment and delight that such a distinguished personage as Lord This or Lady That could even remember anyone so unimportant as he was.

Three cards thrilled him more than all the rest. They came together in the same mail and they brought him the good wishes of Her Royal Highness Princess Alexandra for a happy Christmas.

"I expect you know that not many people get a card from the Princess of Wales written in her own hand," he said to Treves, his eyes looking very moist. "I got three—and every one has a different message!"

Clutching the cards to his breast, he made his way to the crowded mantelpiece and set them in the center, next to the photograph of the Princess. For a long time he stood there, supporting himself with his cane, reading the cards over and over again out loud, as if to convince himself they were real.

Finally it was Christmas Eve. The London was astir with orderlies carrying evergreen trees into the wards and setting them up and merry nurses hanging them with clever decorations. None of the excitement, however, reached as far down as the basement.

Joseph was at his worktable making a basket when Nurse Ireland appeared. In her arms she carried a large bag.

"What do you have there, Nurse?" he fluted, his eyes lighting up.

"That's for me to know and you to wonder about," she replied with a mischievous glance. Reaching into the bag, she drew out long strings of tinsel and streamers of colored paper. "Compliments of Mr. Treves and Nurse Ireland." Climbing up on a chair, she rapidly festooned the room with decorations. Next out of the bag came a handsome evergreen wreath and this she hung in Joseph's window. Holly, with its coral-red berries, came next. By now Joseph was following her about happily, carrying the bag and helping in general.

At length only one thing remained in the bag. He pulled it out. "What's this?" He looked wonderingly at a bunch of forked greenish stems with thick, pale green leaves and waxy white berries.

"Haven't you ever seen that before? A big bloke like you?"

"I've never had much to do with plants, Nurse. What is it?"

"It's mistletoe. We hang it up at Christmastime. If you see a girl you like who's standing under it you may kiss her."

"Oh."

With a bunch of mistletoe in her hand, the pretty young woman walked over to the little Elephant Man. Her bold blue eyes looked directly into his timid brown ones. Raising the mistletoe over her own head, she leaned her round rosy cheek close to his mouth. "You may give me a kiss if you've a mind to."

"Oh." A deep flush flooded the grotesque face. Instinctively, Joseph took a step backward and turned his eyes away.

"Joseph, I see you don't fancy me. I suppose I'm not pretty enough for you."

"Oh no, Nurse. I think you're . . . beautiful. But I . . . I . . ." The bird-voice trailed off in a stammer.

"It's *Christmas Eve*, Joseph." Holding the mistletoe over the little man's head, she puckered her lips and pecked him on his mottled cheek. "Happy Christmas, Joseph, and many more of them." She gave him a quick, tight hug and rustled out of the room. Her perfume lingered behind her.

Joseph dropped into his armchair. For a while he sat motionless. Then his fingertips rose to his cheek, to the spot where she'd pressed her mouth. They rested there a moment. Then they moved to his mouth.

His lips were too twisted and bloated to kiss anyone, but with his tongue he could still taste the sweetness of her on his fingertips.

FIFTEEN

Christmas and Boxing Day

A sharp frost had set in. On Christmas morning Joseph's window was crusted white with crystals. After breakfast he sat listening cozily to the crackling of the fire, gazing at the gay decorations all around his room and remembering who had put them there.

A light tapping broke into his reverie. Before he could get up, his door was thrown open and in trooped five young nurses, their faces flushed and happy. They gave no sign they found the Elephant Man different from any other patient in the hospital.

"Happy Christmas, Joseph!" they giggled. And at once their voices, lively and sweet, filled the small room:

> *"Good King Wenceslas looked out,*
> *On the feast of Stephen,*
> *When the snow lay round about,*
> *Deep and crisp and even;*
> *Brightly shone the moon that night,*
> *Though the frost was cruel,*
> *When a poor man came in sight,*
> *Gathering winter fuel."*

Onward they caroled, to the end of the old song. The little man listened open-mouthed, shaking his head in rapture. Waving good-bye, the nurses hurried out to another ward.

Joseph had hardly settled back in his chair when he was startled by a firm rap on his door. In strode a striking figure dressed in a long red robe. He had a long full white beard and a head of white hair crowned with a wreath of ivy. On his back he carried a heavy, bulging red sack.

"Happy Christmas to you, Merrick," boomed Father Christmas. His voice, in contrast to his white beard and hair, was young and lively. Under the disguise Joseph recognized one of Frederick Treves's house surgeons. Behind the red-robed figure came Treves himself, all smiles.

"Happy Christmas, Doctor. Happy Christmas, Mr. Treves." Joseph couldn't hide his excitement. "What's in that big red sack?"

"Guess what." Laying down the bag, Father Christmas began to empty it. He took out one colorfully wrapped package after another, heaping them on the table. "Whew! You do have a lot of friends." He shook the little man's hand warmly. "It's good to see you looking so well and cheerful, Joseph. God bless you and keep you so. You're a shining example to all of us." He slapped Joseph affectionately on the shoulder. Shaking Joseph's hand again, he left.

Treves eyed the pile of packages. "You are a great popular favorite, Joseph. Why, you've received more gifts than anyone in my house!"

Joseph couldn't open the packages fast enough. Supporting each one with his bulky right hand, he pulled the paper off with the left. "I wonder what's inside," he said, his voice shaking, as he opened the first one. "Why, it's a Bible from the Duke of Cambridge! Just look at the handsome leather binding!" He unwrapped the second. "Here's a Toby mug from Lady Nevill. I think I'll put it on the mantel next to her picture."

"If you can find room for it." The surgeon grinned.

Each gift, after it was opened, was held up for Treves to see and admire, then carefully laid on the floor. Before long Joseph was

113

surrounded by a low wall of presents. It was almost an hour before he came to the last package.

"This one feels very heavy," he said. "What can it be, sir?" He gave Treves a meaningful glance. "Is it . . . ?"

"Is it what? I haven't the slightest notion what you mean, Joseph."

"I wonder."

Eager fingers stripped away the paper. Inside was a dressing case of shining black leather.

"Thank you, thank you, Mr. Treves!" He unlatched the case and exclaimed over its silk lining. One at a time he removed the things inside. Holding them at arm's length, he turned them about and examined them. As he did so he cried out with pleasure.

He came to the silver cigarette case. He held it so it would catch the light from the fireplace. "Beautiful."

"Why don't you open it?"

"Good heavens, it's full of cigarettes! The advertisement didn't say anything about cigarettes. It was you put them in, wasn't it, Mr. Treves? Would you like one?"

"Why, thank you." Treves helped himself to a cigarette and lit it. Joseph took one himself, held it to his nostrils, and sniffed. Placing one end close to his lips, he pretended to puff on it. "Egyptian tobacco, I presume," he said in the tone he imagined a lord in a Mayfair club might use. Then, with a flourish, he put the cigarette back in the case and snapped it shut. Back into the dressing case went every object that had come out of it, each replaced with adoring care.

"I just love my dressing case," said Joseph. "I've wanted one like that for ages."

"There's something else in store for you, my lad—and I don't mean just the turkey and plum pudding coming with Christmas dinner. You do remember saying you wanted to go to the theater?"

"I do, I do! When shall we go? Today? Tomorrow?"

"There's no show on Christmas Day. We're going on Boxing

Day.* Mrs. Kendal has obtained places for us at the Theatre Royal in Drury Lane. They're very good seats—and very private ones too. Nobody in the theater will even know you're there."

Joseph could hardly wait for the night of his excursion to the theater. On Boxing Day he was already looking at his watch early in the afternoon. When Treves finally walked into the basement apartment in the evening, the little man had been waiting in his cloak, his hat on his head, for an hour.

"Joseph, you're to be quite the ladies' man tonight. We're not going to the theater by ourselves. We're to have the company of three attractive young ladies. Nurse Ireland and two other nurses. Do you approve?"

"I don't know what to say, Mr. Treves—except that I'm very happy."

The three nurses were waiting in the hospital lobby. Joseph, used to seeing them in their everyday uniforms and aprons, couldn't get over how splendid they looked in the evening gowns and cloaks they had put on for the occasion. He stammered with delight. They went outside and climbed into a waiting carriage. Treves drew the curtains. The little Elephant Man wasn't going to be the object of any stares or pointed fingers if he could help it!

It was a long ride from the dingy slum streets of Whitechapel to the glitter of the West End and its theater district, but for Joseph the time passed swiftly. Never had the surgeon seen him gayer or more talkative.

As they approached Drury Lane the carriage slowed down. Joseph could hardly stay in his seat when he saw the front of the Theatre Royal, with its sign displaying the words *Puss in Boots* and the figure of a booted cat dressed as a cavalier. A long line of carriages was discharging a stream of excited children and their

---

*Boxing Day, the first weekday after Christmas, is a holiday in Great Britain. It is celebrated by giving Christmas boxes containing gifts to postmen and other service workers.

115

parents. Strangely, the carriage carrying Treves and his party didn't stop but moved slowly on.

"Mr. Treves, Mr. Treves!" cried Joseph anxiously. "We're passing the theater. Please tell the coachman to stop!"

"Don't worry, old man. This is a very special event and so we are privileged to use a very special entrance. Here it is now."

The theater manager was waiting to receive them.

"Ah, Mr. Treves, isn't it? And this must be Mr. Merrick. It's a great pleasure, I'm sure. This is the *royal* entrance, ladies and gentlemen. Please follow me."

He escorted them up a private staircase, where there was no one to gape at Joseph's slow-moving, strangely dressed figure. Although it was the royal staircase, it wasn't the royal box to which he showed them, but it was definitely one of the best in the house, very close to the stage. Its owner, a friend of Mrs. Kendal's, was one of the wealthiest women in England.

"Joseph, you and I will sit at the back," said Treves. "I think the young ladies should have these three chairs in front."

Joseph nodded happily. For the first time in his life he was in the company of three pretty young women and he felt thrilled and honored. Treves saw no need to tell him the principal reason they'd been invited was so they might sit in front and hide him from view. But the three had been good friends to the Elephant Man also, and the surgeon wanted to reward them for their many acts of kindness.

In the dark at the rear of the box Joseph took off his hat and cloak and Treves hung them up.

"Now, Joseph," he said with a smile, "just sit back and enjoy the show like any other gentleman in the house."

But Joseph couldn't sit back or behave like any other gentleman there. He'd never been inside a theater before and everything filled him with astonishment. Leaning forward to get a better view of the theater and the audience, he fluted his pleasure over and over again to Treves and the nurses. Even after the orchestra had struck up the overture he chattered on, bursting with comments, with questions.

The curtain swept upward. The marvelous old tale began to

unfold, the story almost everyone has heard in childhood. In the pantomime it was richly adorned with joyful comic songs and dances, with lavish settings, and was brought to life by dozens and dozens of performers in extravagant costumes. Joseph, his jaw slack, watched as the talking cat (played by a popular young actor) skillfully wove his plot to make his lowly master into a noble marquis and help him win the king's daughter for his wife.

"What a wonderful cat!" exclaimed Joseph breathlessly. "I can hardly wait to see what he does next."

The little man was so swept up in the doings onstage he forgot who he was and where he was. In the excitement he kept bouncing around on his chair; several times Treves had to put an arm around him to keep him from falling off. Joseph was having a good time but the surgeon was having an even better one. He took delight in seeing the delight of his patient.

The pantomime came to a climax. Puss in Boots was confronting a terrible ogre. He challenged the giant to prove he could transform himself, as he claimed he could, into the smallest of animals. By the magic of the theater the ogre became a mouse. In an instant Puss pounced upon him and swallowed him. The theater shook with the children's happy howls. Joseph rocked joyfully from side to side in his seat. Treves and the nurses applauded.

Treves suddenly became aware he was yawning. He took out his watch. Past eleven! His day had been a long one, for he'd risen at 5 A.M., as he always did, to work. Joseph, however, showed not the slightest sign of fatigue or diminishing interest. Even after the last encore had been sung and people were shuffling out of the theater he sat glued to his seat, unwilling to believe his glorious evening was at an end. With the nurses' help Treves managed to shepherd him down the stairs, out of the theater, and back to the waiting carriage without attracting attention.

All the way back to the hospital Joseph was a very different person from the one he had been on the way to the theater. He sat silent, motionless, like a person hypnotized.

But later! For weeks, when Treves dropped in on him, Joseph

117

bombarded him with questions about *Puss in Boots*. It was just about the only thing he wanted to talk about.

"I wonder what the princess did after we left," he said to Treves. Or: "Do you think that poor man is still in the dungeon?" To Joseph, in his childlike simplicity, it wasn't make-believe he'd seen but an episode in real life, and it continued to go on and on after the curtain had fallen. Everything in it was real. The castle was a real castle. The ogre was a real ogre. The princess was of the blood royal. Even the dishes at the banquet had been made of solid gold.

Certain parts of the pantomime he came back to over and over again, perhaps because they touched springs in his own life.

"Oh, Mr. Treves, did I enjoy it," he exclaimed, "when that silly policeman got knocked down and slapped in the face! The police, you know, were always closing down my show in this country. In Belgium too. They didn't treat me very nicely either. Why? I hadn't done anything wicked. All I did was try to earn a living so I wouldn't have to go back to the workhouse. Was that so wrong? . . .

"Oh, that princess!" His eyes rolled upward. "I adored her. Now there was a beauty. But so were the young ladies in the ballet. I could have sat there for hours and hours watching them dance. What long legs they had! What beautiful long legs!"

SIXTEEN

The Journey

Outside Joseph's open window a sparrow burst into song. The little man, weaving a basket, paused to listen.

His door swung open.

"Hallo there, how are you, lad?"

"Can't complain, Mr. Treves, can't complain."

"Good." A friendly hand perched on Joseph's shoulder. "You've often told me how much you'd like to spend some time in the country—"

"Oh, Mr. Treves, it would make me so happy!" He nodded his enormous head toward his overflowing bookcase. "I read about it all the time. You know, I've seen so little of the country. I was city born and bred. I can barely tell a daisy from a dandelion." Sadness edged his voice. "All I know of the country is what I've glimpsed from a show wagon as I was being taken from one town to the next."

Treves smiled a special smile. "You should see a good deal more of it very shortly. You've been looking peaked lately. It will do you good to get away from the London after all these months here. I've arranged for you to spend six weeks at a cottage outside Northampton. On Lady Knightley's estate. The property is heavily wooded and you'll be free to wander about. Do you think you can be packed and ready to leave by nine tomorrow morning?"

"You know I will, sir."

"That's settled, then. Nurse Ireland has agreed to ride down with you to the train and see you aboard. You'll have to travel by yourself but it's not a very long trip. And you're going in style."

"What do you mean, Mr. Treves?"

"You'll find out soon enough. Have a good time, old chap."

The next morning Joseph and Nurse Ireland left the London in a closed four-wheeler with blinds drawn. It was a long time since the nurse had seen her patient in such high spirits.

"Just think!" cried Joseph. "I'll really be living in the country! I've often read about the nightingale's song—and now perhaps I'll be able to hear it. If there are any sheep, maybe I'll be allowed to feed them. There'll be all those wonderful fresh vegetables and fruit on the dinner table. And flowers! I love flowers but I don't really know one from another."

"I love flowers too. Will you bring me a bouquet when you come home from the country?"

"You won't have to ask me a second time, Nurse."

The carriage came to a halt. Joseph lifted the edge of the curtain and looked out.

"Nurse, this isn't the railway station."

"London railway stations are crowded places. Mr. Treves doesn't think you especially enjoy crowds. No, this is a siding some distance away." She pointed to the second-class coach waiting on the track, its curtains drawn. "Joseph, you have influential friends, and they've made special travel arrangements for you with the railway authorities."

"Special travel arrangements? I don't understand."

But Nurse Ireland, who had already begun to climb down from the carriage, didn't hear. Joseph was in such a hurry that he forgot to ask his question again.

The Journey

The cabbie helped Joseph out. Nurse Ireland wanted to give him a hand with his bag but he insisted on carrying it himself to the railway coach.

Standing in the doorway, Joseph waved to Nurse Ireland. "Will you be here to meet me when I come back?"

"You know I will, Joseph." Her eyes crinkled in a smile. "You'll probably forget all about me while you're in the country!"

"Not likely. Don't be surprised if you get a long letter from me every day."

A tall railway guard approached. Saluting, he looked at Joseph with considerable interest. "Best to take your seat, sir." He nodded toward a steam engine that was rapidly drawing close, belching sparks and black clouds of smoke. "That locomotive will push us on toward the station, where we're to couple up with the Northampton train."

Under his mask Joseph blew a kiss to Nurse Ireland. He was glad she couldn't see it. After a long, hard wave he shut the door. He looked up and down the car before taking a seat. So far as he could tell, he was the only passenger. No doubt others would get on when they reached the station.

At the station the coach was linked up to the rear end of the Northampton train. Joseph peered out between the blinds at the platform. Passengers were boarding the other cars. At any moment he expected someone to open the door of his compartment, sit down opposite, and stare at him bug-eyed. Just the thought of it made him shiver. His shoulders hunched up.

But no one came in.

At last the train got under way. It rattled along the glittering tracks, pouring huge white plumes of smoke into the sky. Joseph, still fearful that other passengers might enter, crouched in his corner, clutching his cane and bag.

Abruptly the door to Joseph's compartment clanged open. The big train guard loomed over him.

Joseph looked up, his heart pounding.

The man saluted. "Why don't you take off your hat and cloak, sir, and make yourself at home? You do have the whole coach to yourself, sir. All the way to Northampton. If you need anything at all, just call me. I'll be at the front." He saluted again and left.

The whole coach to himself! Now Joseph understood what Treves had meant the other day when he'd said Joseph would be traveling in style. He could hardly believe his good fortune. So far as he knew, only one person in the entire kingdom had a private coach and that was the Queen.

Sitting in the compartment, listening to the clicking of the wheels on the track, Joseph suddenly remembered his last trip by rail two years before. How different that journey had been! He'd just arrived from Belgium and was on his way to Liverpool Street Station in the boat train. He recalled the coach's drafty corridor and himself standing in it, hungry and exhausted, hour after hour. Shrinking against the wall when someone went past. Not daring to enter a compartment and sit down. Not daring to look at the cold, unfriendly faces of his fellow passengers.

He glanced about his compartment. It had places for seven. The coach had ten compartments. Places for seventy—but he was the only passenger.

Times had certainly changed!

Not his feelings, though. He would always be afraid of trains. He decided to keep his cloak and hat on.

The train chugged past one small station after another. Lifting the curtain, he looked out. Soon smoke-stained factories and warehouses and rows of workingmen's houses gave way to rolling downs of green with, here and there, a little country cottage. Not far off he could see sheep and cattle grazing in the meadows. A mare and her foal looked up and watched the train go by.

The country! How often he'd longed to be there! He was going to have the time of his life!

The train picked up speed. The whistle of the locomotive shrieked in its high-pitched, mournful voice.

The Journey

It was the first time since Joseph had been taken in at the London that he'd left it so far behind. Frederick Treves, Nurse Ireland, all his other friends—his whole snug little world at the hospital—seemed a million miles away.

How terribly alone he felt!

SEVENTEEN

The Mirror

Wheels screeching, the train groaned to a halt. "Northampton!" called the burly guard and hurried toward Joseph to
help him down from the coach. The little man was already on his
feet, cane in one hand, bag in the other.

Nervously he looked up and down the railway platform. He'd
been told an escort would be waiting to meet him. But no one came
toward him. All he saw was passengers leaving the train or rushing
to climb aboard.

Doors slammed. The train whistle blew three sharp blasts. Great
billows of steam poured from the locomotive, and the long line of
cars clattered out of the station. In a few minutes they had become a
toy train in the distance.

Where was his escort? Beneath his mask Joseph felt cold drops of
perspiration forming.

The station gradually emptied. Only Joseph remained—Joseph
and a handful of youths who had been helping passengers with their
luggage. Attracted by the strangeness of the lone figure in the cloak
and mask, they formed a knot close by, pointing and whispering.
His uneasiness grew.

All at once a horse-drawn cart mounted on two high wheels rolled rapidly up to the other side of the platform. Jumping down, the driver hurried toward Joseph.

"Mr. Merrick, isn't it?" He was a large, pleasant-looking older man, his face burned brown by the sun. He was dressed in neat, comfortable country clothes and wore boots.

"Yes, I'm Merrick." Joseph sighed with relief.

The pleasant-faced man didn't quite understand what he said but that made no difference. "I'm Goldby, Tom Goldby, Lady Knightley's gamekeeper. Please forgive me, sir, for being late. There was an overturned carriage on the road and I had to help. I do hope you understand. Come this way, please." He picked up Joseph's bag and led him to the cart.

The knot of curiosity-seekers followed, unwilling to give up the novelty of the day.

"Pay them no mind, sir," boomed Goldby loudly so they would be sure to hear. "Some folks just don't know any better." He scooped up the little man and swung him up into a seat in the cart as easily as if he'd been a child. Then he climbed up in front and in an instant they had left the station behind them.

The pony cart rattled along over the cobblestones of the gray city streets and soon Joseph found himself surrounded by the green of the countryside. It was a clear, sunny day with a few fleecy clouds in the blue sky. Tall old elms and oaks looked down on the newcomer and seemed to rustle a leafy greeting. Birds bounced from branch to branch, singing cheerily.

The little man took a deep breath. London's air was always so heavy with soot and dust. Here the air was clean and sweet and full of the fresh smell of moist earth.

"I say!" he exclaimed. "This *is* the country!"

Goldby grinned and nodded.

The cart swung left into a heavily timbered park and jolted along a narrow lane overarched by lofty branches. It went up a gentle slope until it came to a clearing, where it halted in front of a large, brick farmhouse.

"Here we are, Mr. Merrick," said Goldby. "This is Redhill Farm." Climbing down from the cart, he reached up and, placing his hands on Joseph, lifted him down to the ground.

Goldby took Joseph's bag and the little man began to follow him to the house. He had taken just a few steps when he heard a low, deep-throated growl behind. Startled, he swung himself around.

Facing him stood a great, powerfully built brown dog. The animal must have been three feet high. Sunlight glinted on the fierce-looking teeth in his black muzzle. Enraged eyes fixed on the stranger, the dog growled again.

"Hush up, Nelson, hush up!" cried Goldby. "Is that any way to treat a guest? Off with you—and don't you dare come back till you've learned better manners."

Joseph had turned white to his lips. He'd always liked dogs but he hadn't found himself so close to one in years. And this dog in particular looked so big and threatening. He watched, quaking, as the animal slowly moved off. After retreating about fifty yards the dog stopped and turned, still eyeing the newcomer.

The color had returned to Joseph's cheeks. "Hello there, boy," he called and gave a timid wave.

A bark, hoarse and hostile, was the dog's reply.

"I suppose it's your hat and cloak, or your gait, maybe, that stirred him up so, Mr. Merrick. Nelson's a watchdog, one of the best. A mastiff of the old English breed. You don't see many like him nowadays. He'll be all right as soon as he gets used to you."

The farmhouse door swung open. A short, stout, red-faced woman stood framed in the doorway.

"Here's Mrs. Goldby," boomed her husband amiably. "Molly, say hello to Mr. Merrick."

But the woman said nothing. Instead, with a frown, she examined Joseph's curious garments and posture. Suddenly recollecting herself, she curtseyed and held the door for him.

As Joseph hobbled forward the woman's frown deepened.

It would hardly surprise me, he thought, if she bared her teeth and growled, just like her mastiff.

"Won't you give me your hat and cloak, sir?"

126

Her manner was respectful but there was a sharp edge of distrust to her voice. Very slowly he raised the mask that shielded his face. He saw the color fade from her cheeks.

But it was too late now for him to stop. He jerked the hat off altogether.

"Good Lord!" she shrieked at the top of her lungs. "Good Lord!"

Throwing her apron over her face to keep the horrible apparition from her eyes, she rushed blindly past the Elephant Man. Out of the house she dashed and disappeared into the woods.

Joseph's heart beat wildly. His shoulders hunched up. How many times he had lived through the same awful, painful experience! It was that frightened nurse all over again, the one who had brought him his food that first day at the London and then dropped the tray and ran. It was a hundred other women who had turned away in horror from the sight of him. Yet always, always it felt like the first time.

What a terrible mistake he'd made to leave his safe little home at the hospital!

"Dear me, dear me," Goldby apologized. "I never reckoned she'd carry on this way. I'm so sorry. I should have told her a bit more about you. Believe me, she's a good Christian woman, Mrs. Goldby is. I'm sure she'll come round. Mr. Merrick, you just stay put for a moment or two while I go and explain things to her. Believe me, everything will be fine, just fine." He hurried out, shaking his head.

Dazed, Joseph stood motionless in the empty room. It was large and attractive, with a table and chairs, a big stone fireplace, and over that two fowling pieces. Outside he could faintly hear Goldby calling, "Molly! Molly!"

At the left something glittered and caught his eye. He looked closer.

It was a mirror hanging on the wall.

A good two years had passed since Joseph had last seen a mirror. Any object of the kind had been strictly banned from his basement apartment by Treves. Now, suddenly, there was one close at hand. It both lured the little man and repelled him.

Cautiously he edged over toward it.

Perhaps he wanted to prove to himself that Mrs. Goldby had done him an injustice. Perhaps he'd forgotten how shocking he used to find his face. In the hospital, without a mirror to consult, he had persuaded himself, almost, that he couldn't look as dreadful as he once had thought. Then, too, the people Treves was always introducing him to were so accepting, so complimentary. Couldn't his face have improved . . . a little?

He looked into the glass.

A cry of anguish burst from his lips.

If his face had appeared terrible to him two years earlier, now it seemed a dozen times more monstrous.

The warty growth disfiguring his neck had spread. It had traveled up over his chin, onto his cheek, the back of his head. The pink outgrowth of bone from his upper jaw thrust downward still farther. His twisted mouth was even more twisted than he could remember. His bloated lips seemed to have blown up to twice the size they were before. His chin almost came to a point. The nose looked as if someone had smashed it in.

But the loaf of bone on his forehead! He ran his trembling fingers over it as if for the first time. It was enormous—so enormous that he understood suddenly why his head had been feeling so heavy. He understood why, when he lay down to sleep, his head sank back into the pillow so deep he sometimes felt pressure on his throat, as if he were suffocating. And he had been telling himself it was his imagination!

Never had his face looked so thin and haggard. Or so hideous. It was the face of some monstrous stranger, but a stranger he recognized. Only twenty-six, he thought. I look like a man of sixty or older. And with a loud cry he covered his face with both hands and sobbed.

There was a flurry of footsteps behind him. I must get hold of myself, Joseph told himself, and he did. Turning, he saw Tom Goldby's brown face, a look of concern on it.

"Dear me! The mirror. We were told to take it down. Please excuse me." As Goldby spoke, his big hands rapidly removed it.

"That's that." He cleared his throat. "Mrs. Goldby has something to say to you."

The gamekeeper's wife stepped forward. Her face was pale and stained with tears.

"I beg your pardon, Mr. Merrick," she said with a curtsey. "Honest to God, I can't imagine what came over me. How weak and unchristian! Mr. Goldby has just told me all about you. The Prince and Princess of Wales call you their friend—and I dared to turn my back on you! God forgive me! Poor gentleman, I hope you'll find it in your heart to do so too. You must be tired and hungry. Please give me your cloak and hat and sit down at the table. I'll bring you some lunch at once."

Joseph murmured something, he didn't know what. But her sweetness and honest regret had moved him. His spirits began to revive.

Mrs. Goldby went bustling into the next room—he supposed it was the kitchen—followed by her husband. In ten minutes she was back with a large tray. It held dishes piled high with fresh leafy lettuce, ripe red tomatoes, the greenest of green peppers, cucumbers, yellow cheese, fragrant bread and sweet butter, half a cold pheasant, a mug of tangy apple cider. Country fare! After his long ride in the train and pony cart, food had never looked or smelled so good to Joseph. His misery of a few minutes earlier had somehow whetted his appetite. He fell upon the food as if he hadn't eaten in weeks.

From the kitchen he could hear the clatter of crockery and the hum of low voices. The Goldbys, he judged, were having their own lunch. The noises were comforting. Condemned to spend so much of his life by himself, he liked to hear the sound of people nearby. At the same time he preferred to eat alone, away from the astonished glances and raised eyebrows of the curious and unfeeling.

Behind him Joseph heard a slight sound. He turned his head and looked into the dark eyes of Nelson, the big mastiff. Evidently the outer door had not been shut and the dog had pushed it open and come in. Nelson was glaring at him. Low, menacing noises came from the animal's throat. His body close to the floor, he crept slowly nearer. Was he getting ready to spring?

Somehow, this time Joseph felt no fright. For most of his short life he'd had much more to fear from people than from animals. And he had always been fond of dogs.

"Nelson, Nelson," Joseph called in his high, fluting tones, looking into the dog's eyes, "I want to be your friend."

Nelson's tail sprang erect at the first word. Whether it was the sound of his own name or the special quality of Joseph's voice, the animal stopped growling. His tail began to wag.

"What would you say to a peace offering?" Joseph heaped some food on a dish and set it down on the floor. "Eat it, boy. It's for you."

The mastiff inched forward and sniffed the food. Instantly a piece of meat disappeared down his throat. Then he gulped down another and another until the dish was empty and he had licked it clean. Sitting down on his haunches, he gazed up at Joseph. The distrust was gone from his eyes.

"We will be friends, old boy, won't we?" Joseph ran his hand along the top of the mastiff's head and gently scratched his neck. Nelson narrowed his eyes contentedly. When Joseph stopped patting him, he lifted his head and pushed the top of it against Joseph's hand.

"Want me to pet you some more, boy? Of course I will." He looked into the dark liquid depths of the dog's eyes. "I know my disease is getting worse and it shows. I nearly frightened poor Mrs. Goldby to death. But I don't frighten you at all, Nelson, do I?"

If Joseph had spent a few moments in hell, the next weeks he passed in paradise. Mrs. Goldby showed herself kind and thoughtful in a thousand ways. Her husband quickly came to understand his guest's peculiar speech. Taking time from his duties, he often went on long walks with him in the forest. There he showed the little man what only a woodsman could, the haunts and secret ways of the wild things.

Every day brought new discoveries for Joseph. He met birds he had never seen before and listened to their songs. He sat by the side of a stream and watched the trout as they slipped silently past. He startled a hare and was almost as frightened by it as it was by him. Each experience was an exciting adventure.

Wherever he went he carried a book with him. When he saw a wild flower that took his fancy he plucked it and pressed it between the pages. To anyone but Joseph the flowers might have seemed very commonplace and not worth picking. To the little man, however, every flower was a rare treasure. He loved them the way a small child does—for their colors, their freshness, their fragrance. Almost every day he wrote to Frederick Treves and Nurse Ireland to tell them about the things he had seen and done. After he finished each letter he pressed a flower between its pages. If his friends couldn't share his special holiday, at least he could share his flowers with them.

After six weeks Joseph's visit to Northampton came to a close. He had already thanked his hostess, Lady Knightley, who invited him to come again the following year; now he shook hands warmly with Mr. and Mrs. Goldby and climbed into the special railway car that would carry him home to London.

In just a few hours he was back in the city. As the coach was shunted to the familiar siding, he peered eagerly out the window. A closed four-wheeler was waiting nearby.

His hope was not disappointed. Nurse Ireland hurried over to greet him, and she was even lovelier than he remembered.

"How well you look, Joseph! You've been breathing that good fresh country air, I can tell. It's a pleasure to have my favorite patient back." Her soft blue eyes laughed into his solemn brown ones.

"I hated to leave the country. But now I don't mind at all."

"Why are you holding your hand behind your back?"

"I didn't forget, Miss Ireland! I didn't forget!"

She took the gift he held out to her. It was a very tiny bouquet of wild flowers that he had painstakingly gathered that morning. The heads of some of them were crushed and some had petals missing, and almost all were a little the worse for wear.

"What a beautiful bouquet!" she cried. "And you carried it all the way from Northampton for me." Holding it to her nose, she breathed in its perfume. "They are exquisite." She gave the little man a quick, affectionate hug. "Thank you, Joseph. Thank you very, very much!"

They were almost back at the hospital before he could find his tongue again.

EIGHTEEN

To Sleep Like Other People

Frederick Treves laid the stethoscope down on his desk. "You can put your things on now, Joseph. Your examination is finished."

"How do you find me, Mr. Treves?"

"Well enough, old chap. I was worried about your heart but it's holding up nicely." He paused. "You've been looking rather tired lately."

"I've not been sleeping too well. It must be that funny position I have to sleep in. How I dislike it! But you know all about that."

The surgeon certainly did. Joseph's head had grown so enormous and so heavy, it was no longer safe for him to sleep on his back. If he did, the strain on his neck made him feel he was suffocating. For eighteen months now he'd been sleeping sitting up. Propped up in back with pillows, he slept with his legs drawn up, his arms around them, his head resting upon his knees.

"Perhaps it's the position," said Treves. "But I think you may not be getting enough exercise. You should go out walking in the garden more, now that the weather's so fine. Some mild exercise would be good for your heart as well."

"I will try to get more exercise, Mr. Treves. Thank you very much."

The surgeon jotted down some final notes on the Elephant Man's record. He took special care to hide them from his patient's view. For Treves was writing that Joseph's disease was getting worse at an alarming rate. Every time Treves examined him he found more of his body affected. The flaps of warty skin hanging from his back and shoulder had grown longer and heavier. The tumors continued to spread. The growth from his upper jaw was now so big his speech was becoming difficult even for Treves to understand. Worst of all, his great dome of a head and its bony outcroppings had gotten much larger.

At twenty-seven Joseph looked like a man of seventy-five or more, and he moved about like one.

How much longer could he go on? It was impossible to tell. There were no records of anyone with a disease like Joseph's. But, judging from his appearance, the end could not be far off.

"That's all for now, old chap. Nurse Ireland will see you back to your rooms."

The days were growing longer. It was April and Easter was at hand. Joseph and the chaplain of the London had become good friends; the two sometimes talked together for hours. Joseph, who had become a member of the Church of England, attended the services in the hospital chapel regularly. Not that anyone ever saw him there. The chaplain had arranged for him to sit in the vestry, a small room off the chapel, during the services. There, with his prayerbook in his hand and the door open just an inch or two, he could follow every word that was spoken and take part in the prayers. He loved especially to join in the singing.

Easter Sunday came. Joseph was in his chair in the vestry early. Later the chaplain came to him and gave him communion in private.

"I can't tell you how much this means to me," Joseph told him. "You are a great help to me. Everyone in the hospital is so marvelous. I am happy every hour of the day. What would have become of me without Mr. Treves and the London Hospital? I thank God for His mercy in bringing me to this haven."

As Joseph's condition grew more serious he needed more and more rest. Most days he stayed in bed all morning, not rising until noon.

Friday, April 11, 1890, was one of those days. Every morning Nurse Ireland came in to see how he was. When she pushed open his door that morning he was sitting up in bed, reading.

"Good morning, Joseph. How are you today?"

"I can't complain, Nurse."

"You don't look very comfortable to me. Lean forward now." She straightened the pillows supporting his back. "There, isn't that better?" With a friendly wave of the hand she left.

At 1:30 P.M. the wardmaid came in with Joseph's lunch on a tray. He was still in bed, reading.

"That must be a mighty interesting book, Mr. Merrick."

"It is, Miss. A mighty interesting book." He yawned.

Putting down the full tray, the young woman picked up the one with the remains of his breakfast. The door closed quietly behind her.

Somehow Joseph couldn't bring himself to get up and dress. He felt a bit sleepy. Was it because he'd been up so late last night walking in the garden?

A feeling of warmth and contentment crept through his body. How comfortable I am! he thought. The book slipped from his lap.

He became aware he was moving down in the bed and the pillows were moving down with him, his head resting on one of them.

He knew he shouldn't be doing it.

But he wanted to. It felt so good.

His heavy head sank deeper into the soft pillow.

For an instant he felt a pain in his neck. Somehow he didn't mind it. He almost enjoyed the sensation.

Joseph became drowsier and drowsier. He drifted off to sleep.

A little after three o'clock Treves's young house surgeon, Mr.

Hodges, opened the door to check on Joseph. The little man lay stretched out on his bed. Hodges saw the untouched tray on the table.

"Merrick! Is anything the matter?"

There was no answer.

Alarmed, Hodges ran to the bed. He leaned over and placed his ear against Joseph's chest. He heard nothing.

Hodges rushed out in search of the senior house surgeon, Mr. Ashe. He found him and the two went downstairs.

"He's still warm." Ashe made a brief examination. "But he's dead, sure enough. It was sudden but I can't say it was unexpected. We'd best get in touch with Freddie Treves. Merrick was his favorite patient. He'll want to know at once."

Hodges went out into the afternoon sunshine and jumped into a waiting cab. When he reached 6 Wimpole Street Treves's house was overflowing with patients.

"Poor Joseph! I am sorry. I'll tell Nurse to send the patients home and we'll go back directly."

In the basement room Joseph's body lay just as the surgeons had left it. Ashe and Hodges looked on as Treves made his examination.

"He was such a good sort," said Treves. "I wish I could have done more for him." He took Joseph's head in both hands and turned it from side to side. "It was a dislocation of the neck, I think. He must have gone to sleep with his head lying on the pillow. It's quite soft and his head sank back into it, causing the dislocation."

"Do you suppose he suffered much?"

"I don't think so. The bed isn't disturbed and he looks very calm." Treves stroked the dead man's hand. "Poor Joseph! He wanted nothing in the world so much as to be like other people. He often told me how much he wished he could lie down to sleep like the rest of us." Treves sighed. "This time he must have decided he would."

Afterword

I have had the moving experience of meeting the Elephant Man in person. Not in the flesh, to be sure, but in the bone. In the museum of the London Hospital Medical College Joseph Merrick's skeleton stands, leaning somewhat to the right as the little man did in life, an expression of perpetual surprise on his face of bone. (Things have turned out almost as he predicted. Dr. Wilfred Grenfell, in his autobiography, noted that Merrick often said he expected the hospital would keep his body preserved in a big glass jar of alcohol.) Close by are casts of parts of his body made after death, as well as his great cap and mask and the Gothic cathedral of cardboard he made as a gift for Dame Madge Kendal.

The skeleton of the Elephant Man has been viewed by generations of medical men and women at the London. It is an awesome sight. The spine is curved in an S shape (a severe form of a condition called scoliosis). The bones of the skull are greatly enlarged and deformed, especially the cranium and the lower jaw. The bones of the right arm and leg are also overgrown. The cast of the head, with its glass eyes, seems pathetically lifelike.

An inquest into Joseph's death was held at the London Hospital in April, 1890. It is interesting to note that the body was identified by his uncle, Charles Merrick, who had come to London for the purpose. The inquest report observes that Joseph's father was still alive but does not suggest he was present. Nurse Ireland testified that Joseph was in his usual health when she looked in on him on his last morning. Dr. Ashe, the house surgeon, testified that there were no signs of violence and that he believed Merrick had died of suffocation while asleep; "the weight of the head overcame him." The coroner's jury accepted this view.

Today the disease that Joseph Merrick suffered from is called neurofibromatosis (NF) or multiple neurofibromatosis. The word root *neuro* means *nerve*; a fibroma is a tumor of fibrous tissue. Neurofibromas are tumors that appear in association with the nerves. They may be present on the skin or beneath it, on the bone, or almost anywhere in the body. Other names for the disorder are Von Recklinghausen's disease (for the German doctor who first described NF in detail) and Elephant Man's disease.

Neurofibromatosis, as it existed in Joseph Merrick, was exceptionally severe. His may actually be the most extreme case ever described. The average case of NF bears little resemblance to Merrick's. Sometimes the disease is so mild that it escapes notice. About one hundred thousand Americans have it; every year about one birth in three thousand is affected by it. In the United Kingdom there are some twenty thousand cases of NF. It is one of the commonest of hereditary neurological disorders.

NF is a genetic disease. Usually it is inherited, but it may occur spontaneously by a genetic mutation in an unborn child. Whether Joseph Merrick's case was inherited or spontaneous is impossible to say, since little is known about his parents. It was related that his mother was a cripple. The child of a parent who has NF has a 50 percent chance of inheriting it. As yet no prenatal test has been developed to determine whether an unborn child has the condition.

Usually NF can be identified soon after birth. A common clue is the presence of light brown spots (called café-au-lait spots) on the skin. If a child has six or more of these and each is at least half a centimeter in diameter NF is suspected. The number may increase during childhood. Other common complications of NF in children are scoliosis and learning disability.

The tumors or neurofibromas characteristic of NF may be seen in childhood but usually they do not appear until puberty. As a rule they are benign. In a very small number of cases, however, certain NF tumors may turn cancerous. Obviously, anyone with NF requires regular medical checkups.

In some patients the only symptoms may be the brown spots, so the condition may not be noticed by the untrained eye. Other patients may have lumps or tumors in the skin. These may not be conspicuous and often are hidden by clothing. More serious cases can have such symptoms as enlarged or deformed bones. Curvature of the spine, which Merrick had, is a fairly common symptom. Occasionally NF causes problems with hearing and vision. In severe cases sometimes tumors develop on the brain and spinal cord. It is important to bear in mind, however, that most patients do *not* have severe symptoms and are able to lead completely normal lives.

So far no treatment has been discovered that will cure NF. However, physicians can do much, often, to relieve the symptoms. The use of a back brace or surgery can help in correcting bone problems such as scoliosis. If tumors are painful or conspicuous, they may be removed by surgery (as the tumor in Joseph's mouth was removed in Leicester Infirmary), although sometimes they grow back. Tumors on the optic or auditory nerves can be treated surgically, but not in every case.

In December, 1981, attention was drawn to the case of a young woman in Philadelphia, Lisa H., whom the press called "the Elephant Girl." Determined to improve her appearance, she under-went extensive radical surgery for the removal of tumors and the correction of other defects. The operations, which were numerous, required transfusions of more than four times the amount of blood in her body. By 1984 her appearance had been somewhat improved, though changes still fell short of her hopes. But the case of this courageous young woman is a very severe one.

Research on NF is going on at a number of medical centers in the United States. Scientists are working to develop better methods for the treatment and diagnosis of NF. A section of the National Institute of Health (the National Institute of Neurological and Communicative Disorders and Stroke) is doing research on nerve growth, tumor development, and many other related subjects. Work is also being done to locate the mutant gene that causes the disease.

People with NF may not only have medical problems, but they may have social and emotional ones too, especially a deep feeling of isolation, much as Joseph Merrick did. Like him they may feel a sense of stigma. They may not even be aware of the name of the disorder or that many others have it in the same or different forms. For anyone with NF there are organizations that offer help. Of primary importance is the National Neurofibromatosis Foundation, 70 West 40th Street, New York, NY 10018. Through this foundation patients and their families can learn the facts about the disease and be aided in locating medical, social, and genetic counseling. It also furnishes information to health professionals and supports scientific research on NF. The foundation has helped to set up chapters in a number of states, where patients and their families find support and fellowship. In the United Kingdom the organization's counterpart is LINK, 14 Willow Way, Sherfield on Loddon, Basingstoke, Hants, England.

Readers may be interested in learning something more about the man who played such an important part in the fortunes of Joseph Merrick. Frederick Treves (1853–1923) was one of the most respected and successful surgeons of his day. He was widely known for a number of classic works on surgery and he pioneered in the operative treatment of appendicitis. In 1902 he gained world fame. Edward VII, two days before the date set for his coronation, became violently ill with appendicitis. He still wanted to go to Westminster Abbey and be crowned.

"Sir," said Treves, "if you go to the abbey as you are now, you will arrive a corpse."

The coronation was postponed, Treves operated, and the King's life was saved. Treves was created a baronet soon after. He was also surgeon to Queen Victoria, Queen Alexandra, King George V, and a host of other eminent people.

In 1900, during the Boer War, Treves served in South Africa as a consulting surgeon to the British forces in the field. In World War I he was made president of the War Office Medical Board and helped to found the British Red Cross. He gave up the active practice of surgery at fifty-five, believing that the work called for younger hands. During the last two decades of his life his great energy found an outlet in writing books, mostly about travel, which were widely read. His last work, *The Elephant Man and Other Reminiscences*, was published in 1923. Curiously, he always called Joseph Merrick "John" Merrick in the book; this error was perpetuated in the celebrated play *The Elephant Man* by Bernard Pomerance.

Treves died in Switzerland in 1923. His ashes were buried in his native Dorchester, an event commemorated in a poem by his friend the famous writer Thomas Hardy, who was one of the mourners.

This book is a fictional biography. It is only natural for a reader to want to know how much is fiction and how much biography.

The narrative follows the main events of Joseph Merrick's life as they were related by Sir Frederick Treves and others who were acquainted with the Elephant Man or his case. It also draws upon knowledge brought to light by recent research, especially the impressive work of Dr. Michael Howell and Peter Ford mentioned in the Acknowledgments.

The dates are the actual dates. The major characters—F.C. Carr Gomm, Madge Kendal, Leila Maturin, Tom Norman, Joseph's family, and the rest—were actual people who played in real life essentially the same roles they play here. Minor characters like old Bill and Mr. Quiggers are invented. Nurse Ireland, of course, took care of Joseph in reality, but beyond that her part is imagined. It is not far-fetched, however; most nurses are charitable people, and Joseph, according to Treves, "fell in love with every attractive lady he saw."

Although the main events follow the record, minor incidents and many details have been supplied by me. A few examples: Joseph was an inmate of Leicester Union Workhouse from 1879 to 1884, but what work he did there or what meals he ate I do not know. He did make it clear, however, that he hated the place. For details about life in the workhouse I have drawn upon authentic narratives about other workhouses. Regarding Joseph's visit to Treves's house in Wimpole Street, I have leaned heavily on the surgeon's brief account; although Treves does not mention his wife and daughters, certainly they could have been present. Joseph did stay with the Goldbys in the country and Lady Louisa Knightley's journal suggests there was some difficulty at the start but that it was overcome. Actually Joseph visited the country three times between 1887 and 1889. For the purpose of my narrative it seemed best to compress all three visits into one. The dialogue, of course, is all my own, but frequently it echoes Treves's words or those of others who knew Joseph.

All in all, I have told the Elephant Man's story as honestly as I could, while striving to clothe the bare facts of his life in a convincing garment of reality. Throughout, I have sought to make imagined incidents, details, and dialogue arise naturally out of known events while telling (I hope) an interesting story.

Frederick Drimmer
Norwalk, Connecticut

142

Selected Bibliography

Bland-Sutton, Sir John. *The Story of a Surgeon*. London: Methuen, 1930.

Clarke-Kennedy, A.E. *The London: A Study of the Voluntary Hospital System*. London: Pitman Medical Publishing, 1963.

Drimmer, Frederick. *Very Special People: The Struggles, Loves, and Triumphs of Human Oddities*. New York: Crown Publishers, 1973. Revised edition. New York: Bell Publishing Company, 1985.

Flower, Sir Newman. *Just As It Happened*. London: Cassell & Company, 1950.

Grenfell, Sir Wilfred. *Forty Years for Labrador*. Boston: Houghton Mifflin, 1932.

Halsted, D.G. *A Doctor in the Nineties*. London: Johnson, 1959.

Howell, Michael, and Ford, Peter. *The True History of the Elephant Man*. Revised and illustrated edition. New York: Allison & Busby, 1983.

Kendal, Madge. *Dame Madge Kendal by Herself*. London: John Murray, 1933.

Montagu, Ashley. *The Elephant Man: A Study in Human Dignity*. New York: Outerbridge & Dienstfrey, 1971.

Nordin, R.M. *Through a Workhouse Window*. London: C. Palmer, 1929.

Severo, Richard. *Lisa H.: The True Story of an Extraordinary and Courageous Woman*. New York: Harper & Row, 1985.

Treves, Sir Frederick. *The Elephant Man and Other Reminiscences*. London: Cassell & Company, 1923.